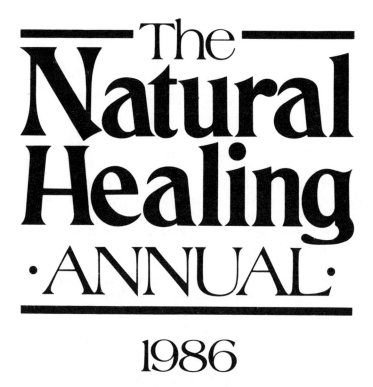

The
Natural
Healing
·ANNUAL·

1986

Edited by
Mark Bricklin
Executive Editor, Prevention® Magazine

Written by the Staff of Rodale Press

Rodale Press, Emmaus, Pennsylvania

ISBN 0-87857-600-2   hardcover
2 4 6 8 10 9 7 5 3 1   hardcover

Contents

Nutritional Healing Newsfront

A Nutritional One-Two against
High Blood Pressure

Two minerals are now believed to be most helpful in
preventing hypertension. Luckily, they're available in
many delicious foods—often together. Here's how to

The Healing Promise of Amino Acids

One of these protein building-blocks seems like a
potent aid for insomnia, and a pretty good
painkiller as well. The others? There's more promise

Are You Safe from B-Vitamin Burnout?

Sometimes the only signal of deficiency is
moodiness, depression or fatigue. Other times,
behavior becomes downright strange. And many
physicians (and friends) have difficulty seeing the

17 Natural Ways to Boost Your Energy

Here are everyday techniques that can add pep to
your step. Diet, work habits, social habits, even
bathroom activities can all work in your favor to help
you get more out of life. Including two great things

Healing That Hernia

Weight, age, heredity and habits can all contribute
to a hernia. But when is surgery really necessary?
What else can be done? Doctors give lots of practical
tips on prevention and control of this common

A Metabolic Perk-Up Plan

New research reveals that many overweight people
eat no more than others. It's their metabolism that's
lazy. Read why, and exactly how to get it moving

Open Your Lungs and Breathe Easy

What can be done to help those who have asthma,
chronic bronchitis or emphysema? This update fills
you in on the advice specialists have concerning
exercise, breathing techniques, nutrition and other

Preventing and Relieving Varicose Veins

Overweight and long standing are two common
triggers. Do you know three others? Support hose
and leg elevation help a lot. Do you know four other
proven helpers? How about the potential benefits
and dangers of different medical treatments? The

Medical Facts to Help You Look Younger

Wrinkles are a major medical and psychological
problem, says a leading dermatologist. Here you'll

New Dimensions in Self-Care

Fitness Newsfront

Practical Psychology Updates

SUPPLEMENTS AND COMMON SENSE

Some of the reports in this book give accounts of the professional use of nutritional supplements. While food supplements are in general quite safe, some can be harmful if taken in very large amounts. Be especially careful not to take more than these commonsense limits:

Vitamin A	20,000 I.U.
Vitamin B_6	50 mg.
Vitamin D	400 I.U.
Selenium	150 mcg.

NOTICE

The information and ideas in this book are meant to supplement the care and guidance of your physician, not to replace it. The editor cautions you not to attempt diagnosis or embark upon self-treatment of serious illness without competent professional assistance. An increasing number of physicians are ready to cooperate with clients who want to improve their diet and lifestyle; if you are under professional care or taking medication, we suggest discussing this possibility with your doctor.

Introduction: The Age of Health Regeneration

Once you make the discovery that the way you live is a more powerful tool than any medical device yet invented, things begin to click.

In this era of the mid-1980s, society as a whole has suddenly made that discovery, and things are going clickety-clack almost faster than you can see.

Everywhere you turn, people are exercising. We're piling our salad bowls higher than ever. We've quit smoking and begun taking our own blood pressures. We're eating high-fiber breakfast cereals and taking calcium supplements. Double martinis seem like a drink left over from the Stone Age; what we're sipping now is mineral water or diet soda with no sugar, no saccharin, no caffeine. State after state is passing seat belt laws and the death and injury toll is diving. Hundreds—perhaps thousands—of businesses have instituted wellness programs to encourage workers to slim down, keep fit and shake off stress.

Bob Rodale, the editor of *Prevention* magazine, calls it Health Regeneration. Regeneration means working to improve what you have, with the resources that are most under your own control. Outside resources are called upon when needed, but the idea is to try to prevent the need for them.

Many physicians are looking at health the same way now, and that's kind of ironic. Think of all the lasers and scanners and computerized analyzers being routinely used today.

But you can scan and compute all day, doctors realize, and never see the payoff—in terms of more healthy people—that you will with lifestyle change. Want to scan something? Try scanning the inside of your refrigerator—or your waistline. Want to compute? Compute how much calcium and beta-carotene and fiber's in your diet. Compute your stress level. Compute your alcohol consumption. Add it all up and you'll find out something about where you stand in this new Age of Health Regeneration.

Neither physicians nor we, the writers and editors of *The Natural Healing Annual,* see any conflict between Regeneration and professional medical care. In fact, they're natural partners.

If you are the take-charge type of person who wants to practice Regeneration, natural healing and other forms of self-help available to you, a physician can be a wonderful resource. Checkups, evaluations, diagnoses and medical advice will all help ensure that your own efforts are going in the right direction, at a safe speed.

The notion that medical care is one thing and natural healing another is no longer true in 1986. More and more physicians realize that it's better to work with nature when seeking health. Even with a serious illness, the self-care, regenerative dimension is being prescribed along with other treatment. It's not a question of medication *or* natural healing, but of How can we reduce—maybe even eliminate—medication by improving lifestyle? . . . How can we improve the outcome of this surgery—maybe even prevent the need for it—by improving lifestyle?

Answers to these questions—in regard to a host of specific health problems—comprise the essence of the 1986 *Natural Healing Annual.* Do keep in mind, though, that no two people are the same, and that what you are about to read is not medical advice but information of a general nature. For personal advice, see your physician. You already know that, I'm sure.

Please enjoy your new 1986 *Natural Healing Annual!*

Mark Bricklin
Executive Editor
Prevention® Magazine

Nutritional Healing Newsfront

A Nutritional One-Two against High Blood Pressure

You might want to go out today and hug a farmer. The prescription to keep your blood pressure down may be growing in his fields and orchards or grazing in his pastures right now.

Potassium, abundant in fresh fruits and vegetables, and calcium, found largely in dairy products, may be science's latest dietary one-two punch in the fight against hypertension.

Recent studies have uncovered what may be an important link between dietary calcium and potassium and blood pressure. Researchers have found that people whose diets are potassium rich—vegetarians, for example—have a low incidence of hypertension even if they're genetically disposed to the condition and don't control their salt intake.

Large population surveys revealed the calcium connection: People with high blood pressure don't seem to get much calcium in the form of dairy products (and it's hard to get much without them). In one test, people who were mildly hypertensive and had lower levels of serum calcium experienced a moderate but consistent drop in blood pressure when they were given oral calcium supplements. The biggest improvement was seen in those people who had the lowest levels of calcium to start with.

The exact mechanisms by which the two essential nutrients regulate blood pressure continue to evade researchers.

1

But both appear to help the body slough off excess sodium and are involved in important functions that control the workings of the vascular system.

Of course, the studies are still new and the evidence is far from voluminous. The calcium theory in particular is still so novel it falls into the hot-controversy category. But even some of the most cautious find it convincing, such as nutritionist Patricia Hausman, author of *The Calcium Bible* (Rawson Associates, 1985). "It's a new idea," says Ms. Hausman. "There aren't a lot of studies, as there are on sodium. I'd call it preliminary but promising. The data there is impressive. I'm leaning toward thinking there's some effect here."

For people who are used to the no-no diets for hypertension, the studies are promising in another way. "The thing that's nice about potassium and calcium is that they're positive nutrients, things people should eat more of," says Arlene Caggiula, Ph.D., associate professor of nutrition at the University of Pittsburgh Graduate School of Public Health. Dr. Caggiula's research focuses on dietary approaches to hypertension, and she has designed well-balanced diets for people with high blood pressure and education programs to help them stick to them. "With sodium you're saying to people, 'You can't eat it.' With potassium and calcium you're saying, 'You can and you should.' "

The other nice thing about potassium and calcium is that they're easy to swallow. Not only is it relatively easy to work these two pressure-lowering nutrients into your menu, you can get them—deliciously—in the same dish. In fact, you can virtually build a diet around the foods they're in. All it takes is a little knowledge and a lot of ingenuity.

Getting potassium isn't tough. "It's in almost everything," says Ms. Hausman. It's abundant in foods that are wonderful for you: fruits, vegetables, beans, fish, poultry and lean cuts of meat.

Getting calcium is not quite as easy. Unfortunately, the foods that contain the most calcium tend to contain a fair amount of fat and sodium, too, which can spell trouble for hypertensives on fat- and salt-controlled diets. However, difficult does not mean impossible. There are plenty of low-fat, low-sodium dairy alternatives—and some calcium-rich foods that haven't even been near the barnyard.

If you aren't hypertensive, by all means don't scratch milk and milk products off your shopping list. "For people to avoid milk because of sodium—unless you have hypertension—is not a good idea," says Leonard Braitman, Ph.D., a statistical consultant who worked on early calcium and hypertension studies. "For some people, like the lactose intolerant, it's not a good food. For other people, it's hard to beat. It's hard to make up your calcium intake with other foods. People should be aware that for people who have hypertension, sodium is a problem. But for others it's probably not."

Ready to start a diet that may last—and lengthen—a lifetime? The first rule of all good menu planning is to make a list. We've done that for you. Save the accompanying lists of potassium- and calcium-rich foods to help you design your own hypertension diet.

● The first thing to do is to exercise your ingenuity. When you take a look at the lists, let your mind start combining familiar foods: yogurt and bananas; salmon fillet with potatoes and broccoli; raisins and nuts. Imagine half a cantaloupe filled with a scoop of ice milk or ricotta cheese. Think about a cooler made in the blender from orange juice, bananas and nonfat dry milk. Before you crack open a cookbook, experiment with your own combinations.

● Armed with your lists, go to the library and look for low-calorie, low-fat and low-sodium cookbooks. Regular cookbooks are fine if you're the kind of inventive chef who knows how to substitute low-fat products for high-fat ones and doctor high-sodium recipes so the taste doesn't vanish with the salt. If you're not, your best bets are cookbooks whose authors have controlled the amount of fat, calories and sodium in their recipes. You'll probably find enough recipes combining calcium and potassium foods to write another cookbook. We did, and here are a few of the books we used.

The Calcium Bible, by Patricia Hausman (Rawson Associates, 1985)

Craig Claiborne's Gourmet Diet, by Craig Claiborne (Ballantine Books, 1981)

The Complete Low-Sodium/Low-Salt Cookbook, by Edith Tibbetts and Karin Cadwell (Sterling Publishing Co., 1984)

Healthy Cooking, by Sharon Claessens (Rodale Press, 1984)

Cooking with Fruit, by Marion Gorman (Rodale Press, 1983)

Natural Weight Loss, by the editors of *Prevention* magazine (Rodale Press, 1985).

FOOD SOURCES OF CALCIUM

Food	Portion	Calcium (mg.)
Swiss cheese	2 ounces	544
Yogurt, low fat	1 cup	448
Provolone cheese	2 ounces	428
Monterey Jack cheese	2 ounces	424
Cheddar cheese	2 ounces	408
Muenster cheese	2 ounces	406
Colby cheese	2 ounces	388
Brick cheese	2 ounces	382
Sardines, Atlantic, drained solids	3 ounces	372
American cheese	2 ounces	348
Ricotta cheese, part skim	½ cup	337
Milk, skim	1 cup	302
Mozzarella cheese	2 ounces	294
Milk, whole	1 cup	291
Buttermilk	1 cup	285
Limburger cheese	2 ounces	282
Ice milk, soft serve	1 cup	274
Salmon, sockeye, drained solids	3 ounces	220
Ice cream	1 cup	176
Ice milk	1 cup	176
Pizza, cheese	⅛ of a 14-inch pie	144
Blackstrap molasses	1 tablespoon	137
Soy flour	½ cup	132

● Not only can you get potassium and calcium in the same dish, you can get them in the same food. Here are a few of the foods that are high in both nutrients: sardines, scallops, skim milk, broccoli, salmon, buttermilk, whole milk, soybeans, blackstrap molasses, navy beans, almonds, ice milk and yogurt. If you're exercising your ingenuity, you can probably plan a whole meal—literally from soup to nuts—using just a few of these double-duty foods.

FOOD SOURCES OF CALCIUM
— *Continued*

Food	Portion	Calcium (mg.)
Soybeans	½ cup	131
Tofu	3 ounces	109
Scallops, steamed	3 ounces	98
Broccoli, cooked	½ cup	89
Almonds	¼ cup	83
Chick-peas, dried	¼ cup	75
Collards, cooked	½ cup	74
Dandelion greens, cooked	½ cup	73
Parmesan cheese	1 tablespoon	69
Shrimp, raw	3 ounces	54
Mustard greens, cooked	½ cup	52
Navy beans, cooked	½ cup	48
Kale, cooked	½ cup	47
Broccoli, raw	1 cup	42

SOURCES: Adapted from
Composition of Foods, Agriculture Handbook No. 8, by Bernice K. Watt and Annabel L. Merrill (Washington, D.C.: Agricultural Research Service, U.S. Department of Agriculture, 1975).
Composition of Foods: Dairy and Egg Products, Agriculture Handbook No. 8-1, by Consumer and Food Economics Institute (Washington, D.C.: Agricultural Research Service, U.S. Department of Agriculture, 1976).
Nutritive Value of American Foods in Common Units, Agriculture Handbook No. 456, by Catherine F. Adams (Washington, D.C.: Agricultural Research Service, U.S. Department of Agriculture, 1975).
USDA Nutrient Data Research Branch.
The Calcium Bible, by Patricia Hausman (New York: Rawson Associates, 1985).

● Stock up on low-fat yogurt. "It's a real bonanza food," says Dr. Caggiula. Not only is it low in fat and relatively low in sodium, it's high in calcium and potassium and can be used for everything from salad dressing to dessert. "Plain low-fat yogurt alone has 350 milligrams of potassium, and flavored low-fat yogurt has an average value of 450 milligrams," says Dr. Caggiula. "The best thing is, the low-fat is even higher in potassium than regular yogurt." For high amounts of calcium, look for low-fat

FOOD SOURCES OF POTASSIUM

Food	Portion	Potassium (mg.)
Potato, baked	1	844
Avocado	½	602
Blackstrap molasses	1 tablespoon	585
Yogurt, low fat	1 cup	573
Raisins	½ cup	545
Sardines, Atlantic, drained solids	3 ounces	501
Flounder	3 ounces	498
Orange juice	1 cup	496
Soybeans, cooked	½ cup	486
Banana	1 medium	451
Apricots, dried	¼ cup	448
Squash, winter, cooked	½ cup	445
Cantaloupe	¼	413
Milk, skim	1 cup	406
Scallops, steamed	3 ounces	405
Sweet potato, baked	1	397
Navy beans, cooked	½ cup	395
Salmon, fillet, fresh, cooked	3 ounces	378
Great Northern beans	½ cup	374
Buttermilk	1 cup	371
Milk, whole	1 cup	370
Cod	3 ounces	345
Beef liver	3 ounces	323
Apricots, fresh	3	313
Sirloin, trimmed of fat	3 ounces	307
Round steak, trimmed of fat	3 ounces	298
Haddock	3 ounces	297
Salmon, sockeye, drained solids	3 ounces	293

yogurt to which the manufacturer has added nonfat milk solids, suggests Patricia Hausman. It adds considerably more calcium and no more fat. She also suggests "dressing up" plain yogurt with potassium-rich foods such as frozen orange juice concentrate, raisins, sliced fresh fruit or shredded raw vegetables. If you're not a yogurt fan, you can get all its benefits by hiding it in blender shakes with fresh fruits and a sweetener such as honey or aspartame or in cold fruit soups.

FOOD SOURCES OF POTASSIUM
— *Continued*

Food	Portion	Potassium (mg.)
Pork, trimmed of fat	3 ounces	283
Almonds, toasted	¼ cup	275
Leg of lamb, trimmed of fat	3 ounces	274
Ice milk	1 cup	265
Turkey, light meat, cooked	3 ounces	259
Tomato, raw	1	254
Perch	3 ounces	243
Tuna, drained solids	3 ounces	225
Chicken, light meat, cooked	3 ounces	210
Shrimp, raw	3 ounces	187
Broccoli, cooked	½ cup	127

SOURCES: Adapted from
Nutritive Value of American Foods in Common Units, Agriculture Handbook No. 456, by Catherine F. Adams (Washington, D.C.: Agricultural Research Service, U.S. Department of Agriculture, 1975).
Composition of Foods: Dairy and Egg Products, Agriculture Handbook No. 8-1, by Consumer and Food Economics Institute (Washington, D.C.: Agricultural Research Service, U.S. Department of Agriculture, 1976).
Composition of Foods: Poultry Products, Agriculture Handbook No. 8-5, by Consumer and Food Economics Institute (Washington, D.C.: Science and Education Administration, U.S. Department of Agriculture, 1979).
Composition of Foods: Fruits and Fruit Juices, Agriculture Handbook No. 8-9, by Consumer Nutrition Center (Washington, D.C.: Human Nutrition Information Service, U.S. Department of Agriculture, 1982).
Composition of Foods: Vegetables and Vegetable Products, Agriculture Handbook No. 8-11, by Nutrition Monitoring Division (Washington D.C.: Human Nutrition Information Service, U.S. Department of Agriculture, 1984).

● You can double your calcium intake by using some of Ms. Hausman's ingenuity. Like the dairy folks, you can add nonfat milk solids to dishes simply by adding nonfat dry milk. Two tablespoons of nonfat dry milk added to half a glass of skim milk boosts the calcium from 150 milligrams to 255 milligrams. Add a banana, as Ms. Hausman does in her Banana Smoothie, and you've got a supercharged potassium/calcium breakfast.

To make a Banana Smoothie, combine ¾ cup of skim milk, ¼ cup of nonfat dry milk, ½ tablespoon of peanut butter, a very ripe banana, one to two packets of aspartame or 1 tablespoon of honey and two ice cubes in a blender and process until smooth. One caveat: Though low in fat and sodium, this delicious blender drink is high in calories—282 per serving. If you're dieting, it's not the best snack or thirst quencher, but it's a great and nutritious breakfast or lunch.

When adding nonfat dry milk to milk products, Ms. Hausman uses these proportions; 2 tablespoons milk powder to ½ cup milk; ¼ cup milk powder to 1 cup milk; 6 tablespoons milk powder to 1½ cups milk; and ½ cup milk powder to 2 cups milk.

● While cottage cheese and fruit may be a favorite summer lunch, you can substantially increase the amount of calcium in the meal by substituting ricotta. Though it also has more fat and calories than cottage cheese, ricotta has about 257 milligrams of calcium in ½ cup, compared to only about 80 milligrams in cottage cheese. You can cut out some fat by using part-skim ricotta or by mixing it with low-fat cottage cheese. It's great with high-potassium vegetables, too.

● Try a stir-fry pizza. Make your own pizza dough—or buy it ready-made—but don't turn for the usual toppings. Vegetables like carrots, onions, peppers and broccoli (which is also high in calcium), either stir-fried in a bit of oil or steamed, take the place of tomato sauce. Top with part-skim mozzarella and bake as usual.

● Try canned pink salmon. Salmon is high in potassium and calcium—because of the tiny bones you can eat—and mixes well with cheese and vegetables. Served hot with vegetables or as the star of a cold vegetable-pasta salad, salmon can become a staple of your blood-pressure diet.

● If you have to restrict your dairy intake, soy foods such as tofu and some cooked beans can provide a modest amount of calcium. Tofu in particular can be used in place of cheese in many dishes. It has about 150 milligrams of calcium per four-ounce serving. And it now comes packaged and tasting just like that summer treat, ice cream.

● Though high in cholesterol, shrimp is a fair source of calcium and a delicious ingredient of a vegetable stir-fry high in potassium.

The Healing Promise of Amino Acids

Amino acids. Only a few years ago, they were a ho-hum group of nutrients with an important but unspectacular role to perform as the "building blocks" of protein. Numbering 22 in all, 9 of them were deemed *essential* because our bodies can't make them—we have to glean them from our food.

That was yesterday. Today, those same tame amino acids are the hottest products on the food-supplement shelf. They've been dubbed "the nutrients of the 80s" and "medical foods," and a recent wave of publicity about their reputed powers has sent the public thronging to buy them in unprecedented quantities.

Is such a trend justified? Perhaps. Several highly respected researchers have been revealing the benefits of amino acids for over a decade, and recent work by others shows that high doses of amino acids may have an effect on hard-to-treat diseases like Parkinson's disease and herpes.

Others urge caution, saying that the public should be wary of these admittedly expensive substances until more is known about their side effects. Even those who promote amino acids say that it might still be too early to use them in large quantities without medical supervision. Here's a rundown on the most frequently discussed amino acids and some examples of their benefits and risks.

Tryptophan ● Of all the essential amino acids, tryptophan is the one that is scarcest in the American diet and, at the same time, the one most investigated by nutrition researchers. A number of scientists feel that it has promise as a safe and effective nondrug remedy for insomnia and pain.

Under experimental conditions, tryptophan in doses of one gram or more has been shown to be most effective for people who suffer from *mild* insomnia and for those who take a long time to fall asleep every night. Apparently it takes the body 45 to 60 minutes to turn tryptophan into serotonin, the brain chemical (a neurotransmitter) responsible for tryptophan's effects.

Tryptophan may also be a natural painkiller, and the dentist's chair is one place where it may prove useful. The pain of a root canal operation is significantly reduced, according to one study, if the patient takes tryptophan supplements during the 24 hours preceding the procedure. Researchers at Temple University in Philadelphia were impressed that tryptophan worked without producing the side effects associated with other anesthesia or analgesics (*Oral Surgery and Oral Medicine,* October, 1984).

In the dose levels used in most of these trials, tryptophan appeared to be free of side effects. In the root canal study, patients were asked to take six doses of 500 milligrams each, spaced over 24 hours. In a separate study that involved facial pain, volunteers took three grams of tryptophan a day for four weeks and experienced relief. One to three grams a day seems to be the range most commonly suggested by researchers.

If you use tryptophan, take it between meals with a low-protein food such as fruit juice or bread. Tryptophan can be thought of as the smallest child at a boardinghouse table—the other amino acids (which would be present in a high-protein meal) tend to crowd it out and prevent it from reaching the brain.

Tyrosine ● If we can call tryptophan the anti-insomnia amino acid, then we can call tyrosine the antistress amino acid.

When certain laboratory mice are placed under physical or emotional stress, they stop probing their environment, poking their way through mazes or sitting up on their haunches to look around. But if those mice are supplemented with tyrosine before being exposed to stress, they don't lose their natural inquisitiveness. Their bodies apparently convert tyrosine into norepinephrine, a brain neurotransmitter that is known to be depleted by stress.

Do these findings apply to people? Yes, says Richard Wurtman, Ph.D., of MIT, the experiment's author. "Supplemental tyrosine may be useful therapeutically in people exposed chronically to stress," he says. The catch, however, is that only those people who are under stress would receive a boost from tyrosine. "We did not observe behavioral effects when unstressed rats were given tyrosine," Dr. Wurtman adds (*Brain Research,* volume 303, 1984).

Tyrosine may also help fight depression, or at least magnify the effects of antidepressant medication. One of Dr. Wurtman's depressed patients "improved markedly" after two weeks of tyrosine therapy, and her symptoms returned within a week after she stopped taking the supplements.

Although individual needs may vary, Dr. Wurtman considered 100 milligrams per kilogram of body weight per day an optimal dose. That works out to be about 5,400 milligrams (5.4 grams) of tyrosine a day for someone who weighs 120 pounds. In the experiment above, the supplement was divided into three separate doses each day (*Journal of Psychiatric Research,* vol. 17, no. 2, 1982/83).

One thing to keep in mind: Don't take a supplement of valine, another essential amino acid, when you take tyrosine. Valine may block tyrosine's entry to the brain.

Parkinson's disease may also respond to tyrosine supplementation, though the evidence is weak. By a series of biochemical reactions, the body can turn tyrosine into dopamine, a vital neurotransmitter that Parkinson's patients are usually low in. The tyrosine seems to work best when the disease is still in its mild, early stages (*Neurology,* April, 1981).

Lysine ● Few people had ever heard of this amino acid before it was publicized in the late 1970s as a natural remedy for cold sores, shingles and genital herpes. Because there was, and still is, no safe or effective over-the-counter treatment for herpes (though there are numerous folk remedies), lysine continues to be popular with those so afflicted—especially those people who suffer frequent attacks.

The theory behind lysine supplementation is this: Researchers discovered in the 1950s that the herpes virus can't survive without a diet of arginine. Arginine, like lysine, is an amino acid, one that is plentiful in nuts, seeds and chocolate. Researchers also discovered that lysine competes with arginine, somehow elbowing it out of the way and making it inaccessible to the herpes virus. If lysine could prevent arginine from reaching the virus, the theory went, it could prevent the viruses from multiplying and setting off an active infection.

In a study published in 1983, a group of researchers polled over 1,500 people who had purchased lysine. Among those polled (whose average daily intake of lysine was over 900 milligrams), 88 percent said that the amino acid had indeed helped them. Lysine, they said, seemed to reduce the severity of their attacks and accelerated the healing time (*Journal of Antimicrobial Chemotherapy,* vol. 12, 1983).

These results have been disputed, however, by scientists who attributed them to the placebo effect. University of Miami researchers found that when they gave sugar pills to herpes sufferers and told them it was lysine, most of the patients reported an improvement. The same researchers found that 1,200 milligrams of lysine a day failed to help those people with severe, frequent herpes episodes (*Archives of Dermatology,* January, 1984).

Glutamine ● If you know someone with an alcohol problem, you might ask him or her to try this little-known amino acid, which just might help them recover from their addiction.

Twenty-five years ago, nutritionist Roger J. Williams, Ph.D., wrote a book called *Alcoholism: The Nutritional Approach* (University of Texas Press). The regimen that he recommended for alcoholics included supplements of glutamine, one of the nonessential amino acids. Dr. Williams claimed that glutamine reduces the usually irresistible craving for alcohol that recovering drinkers almost inevitably encounter.

Many authorities on alcoholism reject the very notion that a "sobriety nutrient" exists. But others say glutamine seems to help.

"I've been using a combination of glutamine, vitamin C and niacinamide, 500 milligrams of each, one to three times a day," says Harry K. Panjwani, M.D., a Ridgewood, New Jersey, psychiatrist and a former member of the Advisory Committee of the National Council on Alcoholism. "We don't know how it works. We can only say that somehow the craving is gone. We've used it extensively and the findings have been the same in every case."

Dr. Panjwani isn't alone. Jerzy Meduski, M.D., Ph.D., a professor at the University of Southern California and a member of the task force for nutrition and behavior in Los Angeles County, also tells us that he has had success with glutamine. "The craving for alcohol seems to be the effect of an imbalance in nutrition," he says. "There is no doubt that there is a positive response to nutritional supplementation."

Valine, Isoleucine and Leucine ● Maybe not today, or even tomorrow, but at some point in the future these three amino acids may become the favorite nutrients of aspiring young Arnold Schwarzeneggers. At least one group of body builders in California is experimenting with a combination of the three as an alternative to dangerous anabolic steroids for the purpose of increasing muscle mass.

"There is a theoretical basis for this, but finding the right ratio between the three has been very tricky," says Robert Erdmann, Ph.D., of San Jose, California. "Some people claim they are getting good results with it. You won't see the same dramatic results that you get with steroids, but this is a potentially safer and saner approach."

Although amino acids are already being advertised in weight-lifting magazines, their safety in large amounts hasn't been established. "We don't want to mislead people," Dr. Erdmann told us. "Our research is in its infancy."

Cysteine ● Much has been made of the curative powers of this amino acid, which the body synthesizes on its own. While the hype has been heavy and solid proof scarce, there is some evidence that cysteine (not to be confused with cystine) has certain therapeutic value as a nutritional supplement.

H. Ghadimi, M.D., chairman of the nutrition committee at Nassau County (New York) Medical Center, uses cysteine supplements to treat his patients who are extremely overweight. He contends that there is a link between obesity and the overproduction of insulin, and that cysteine supplements—500 milligrams taken along with vitamin C at the end of a meal— somehow neutralize some of the excess insulin, which is responsible for fat production.

Dr. Ghadimi is enthusiastic about cysteine. "Cysteine is an anticancer, antiaging amino acid," he says, "because it acts as an antioxidant." Like vitamin C, he claims, cysteine protects the body from damage by oxidants—destructive molecules also known as free radicals.

Other researchers have looked to cysteine as a natural shield against the toxic effects of tobacco and alcohol. Or, more specifically, as a shield against acetaldehyde, a dangerous metabolite of alcohol metabolism and a toxic component of cigarette smoke. In animals cysteine has been tested for that purpose in combination with thiamine and vitamin C (*Agents and Actions*, vol. 5, no. 2, 1975).

Arginine and Ornithine ● The recent best-seller *Life Extension*, by California health consultant Durk Pearson and Sandy Shaw (Warner Books, 1982), advised readers to fight the symptoms of advancing age by taking large supplements—several grams or more a day—of these two nonessential amino acids. But extravagant claims made for these two nutrients are not fully substantiated.

In their book, which helped spark the new wave of interest in amino acids, the authors argue that arginine and ornithine can help people lose weight and put on muscle by triggering the release of growth hormones. They also claim that the two amino acids can help prevent cancer by enhancing the immune response.

But doctors don't necessarily agree with these claims. In fact, arginine and ornithine supplements may not be safe if they *do* work as advertised.

"If arginine and ornithine work—if they do raise growth hormone levels—then people shouldn't use them," says Alan Gaby, M.D., a Baltimore doctor who uses nutrition in his practice. "Elevation of growth hormone levels can cause diabetes," Dr. Gaby says. "The bottom line is that there is no solid research on the effects of arginine and ornithine, and I would like to see more studies on their safety before I would tell anyone to take them."

Safety Is the Bottom Line

The "bottom line," as Dr. Gaby puts it, is safety. Until more is known about the safety of amino acids, they shouldn't be used for the self-treatment of serious illness. At the same time, they shouldn't be taken in large amounts for long periods, for any reason.

But many of those who are researching amino acids feel that it is only a matter of time before the benefits of these nutrients are fully appreciated. They believe that amino acids may eventually replace certain drugs in the treatment of diseases such as those mentioned here and potentially many others.

"The potential for amino acids is grand," one researcher told us, and another said with confidence, "In the field of nutritional supplements, amino acids are the new frontier."

Are You Safe from B-Vitamin Burnout?

Aunt Mary wasn't all that old when her husband died—only 65—but in the past 3 years it seems as though she's aged 20, at least as far as her mind goes. She's forgetful, irritable and tired. And some days she's so confused it's heartbreaking. You hate to think she's becoming senile, but what else could it be?

Teenagers are supposed to be rebellious, it's true, but you're beginning to wonder if your 14-year-old daughter's moodiness and hyperactivity aren't above and beyond normal adolescent turmoil. You're also wondering how anyone can live on french fries and soft drinks, which are about the only foods she'll eat these days. Could that be part of the problem?

The divorce was hard on Tim, but he was determined to pick up and go on with his life. Instead, though, he began feeling so emotionally and physically exhausted he found it hard to do his job, much less look after himself. Instead of slowly getting better, Tim is slowly getting worse and worse. Could the stress be catching up with him?

Nutrition-oriented doctors see these kinds of cases again and again, in different combinations of the same factors— aging, long-term stress, poor eating habits, even special metabolic needs. They also see the unfortunate consequences. Aunt Mary could end up in a nursing home before her time; that wall-climbing teenager might become a high-school dropout; and perhaps Tim will find himself severely depressed, even suicidal.

But all three shared a common problem—a B-complex vitamin deficiency. And they all could have gotten relief from their mental woes, perhaps prevented them altogether, if they'd been getting enough of these nutrients to meet their personal needs.

Over the Brink

"Take someone who's just a little depressed or a little stressed because of things going on in his life. That person might find himself eating poorly. And that could lead to nutritional deficiencies that push him over the brink, into true depression or mental problems," says Charles Tkacz, M.D., medical director of the North Nassau Mental Health Center in Manhasset, New York. The center's specialty is finding and correcting nutritional deficiencies in psychiatric patients, an aspect of treatment that's all too often overlooked in traditional medical care.

Robert Picker, M.D., a Walnut Creek, California, psychiatrist, agrees. "I've run into this kind of situation too many times to count," he says. "The body's nutritional needs are increased during times of stress. What may normally be adequate suddenly becomes a deficiency. And that deficiency could begin a vicious circle of mental symptoms that the person just doesn't seem to be able to shake. In fact, as a psychiatrist, I am painfully aware that many of these people are in psychotherapy for long periods of time without ever realizing that the correction of a nutritional deficiency could have significantly helped or possibly cured their problem, or perhaps have prevented it in the first place."

Overall nutrition is essential, but doctors should take a special look at the B-complex vitamins, especially B_6, B_{12}, thiamine, niacin and folate. They've more than earned their reputation as the "antistress" nutrients.

Why are the B vitamins important for our mental health? The brain, it seems, is more sensitive to fluctuations in dietary nutrients than neurologists once thought. It has a special need for B vitamins to perform at its best.

The role of B vitamins is extensive and complex. They are co-enzymes, or catalysts, in many of the body's most basic functions, including the process of oxidation, or the body's burning of food to provide fuel. What this means is that they're needed to supply the brain with its energy source, glucose. Without enough glucose, the brain begins to perform poorly. Fatigue, depression, even hallucinations, can be symptoms of a low glucose level in the brain. B_6 and niacin are the B vitamins most involved in this process.

But the B vitamins play a second crucial role in our mental health. Several are known to be involved in the production of neurotransmitters, biochemicals that allow the brain cells to pass messages along their nerve pathways.

"B_6 is needed for the production of serotonin, a major neurotransmitter in many body functions," says Eric Braverman, M.D., of the Princeton Brain Bio Center in Skillman, New Jersey. "Folate helps produce catecholamines, which control many body functions. B_{12} is needed to produce acetylcholine, another neurotransmitter. In other words, all the chemicals produced by the brain cells depend on nutrients taken into the body, and in many cases, they seem to depend on certain B vitamins."

Working Backward

What happens when they're not there?

"We know that people who aren't getting enough of these nutrients get a whole host of psychiatric and neurological symptoms, like depression, confusion, fatigue and psychosis," Dr. Tkacz says.

It was seeing that volunteers deprived of B_{12} soon sunk into a funk, that prisoners of war fed thiamine-poor polished rice lost muscle coordination and reasoning power, and that diets short on B_{12} or folate could cause symptoms of senility or psychosis that led doctors to begin thinking backward. If nutrient deficiencies caused such problems, perhaps people with these symptoms could be helped with doses of the nutrients they seemed to be missing.

That's exactly what doctors like Tkacz, Braverman and Picker are doing. "We take blood samples for special nutritional testing, then initially put most patients on therapeutic doses of many nutrients, including 40 to 50 milligrams a day of all the B vitamins," Dr. Tkacz says. When the nutritional tests have been evaluated, the patient may be given more of a specific vitamin, mineral or amino acid that's been found to be lacking in his body.

"We've found, and studies confirm, that many depressed patients are low in B_6," Dr. Tkacz says. "A certain number are helped to recover from their depression by taking B_6 under medical supervision."

Derrick Lonsdale, M.D., a Cleveland physician with a special interest in biochemistry and nutrition, found that some of the first signs of a thiamine deficiency were changes in behavior—neurotic symptoms like depression, insomnia, chest pain and chronic fatigue. All 20 of the patients he studied improved with additional thiamine.

Not incidentally, these nervous patients also had poor diets. They were eating lots of "empty calories," usually refined carbohydrates or sugar-laden drinks, foods that used up their thiamine reserves without putting any back, Dr. Lonsdale reports.

And several doctors are looking into folate deficiency as a

cause of depression, insomnia, irritability, forgetfulness and some supposedly psychosomatic disorders.

In reviewing medical literature, A. Missagh Ghadirian, M.D., of the Royal Victoria Hospital, Montreal, found folate-deficiency depression in people taking medications for rheumatoid arthritis, antibiotics, birth control pills and anticonvulsants. "Sometimes the deficiencies are quite severe, but sometimes they are more marginal and might even escape notice," he says. "If the depression is due to deficiency, making sure the patient gets enough additional folate works well to relieve the condition."

Doctors are realizing now, too, that sometimes the first sign of a B_{12} deficiency can be bizarre mental misfirings that resemble psychosis or senility. One 47-year-old woman who had been "seeing" flying saucers was found to have low B_{12} levels. Four days after starting B_{12} supplementation, her hallucinations were gone (*American Journal of Psychiatry,* February, 1983).

One of Dr. Tkacz's recent patients was a confused, forgetful woman in her early sixties. She'd been diagnosed as senile, but her family had decided to check for a nutritional deficiency. It turned out the woman had a very low level of B_{12}, and with just a few injections she recovered completely, Dr. Tkacz says. She'll have to have B_{12} injections for the rest of her life, but that's certainly better than being prematurely consigned to a nursing home.

"A lot of families would have simply written off her symptoms as part of aging, but that's not usually the case," Dr. Tkacz says. "That's why it's so important to be careful when you're dealing with a possible diagnosis of dementia or Alzheimer's disease. You want to make sure you're not dealing with a B_{12} or folate deficiency. I'd say 5 to 10 percent, easily, of elderly people with mental problems really have nutritional deficiencies, and many involve the B-complex vitamins."

"Tea and Toast" Syndrome

It's the borderline B vitamin deficiencies that are most likely to slip through the cracks of traditional medicine—those that might present themselves only as depression, fatigue, irritability—symptoms for which most doctors would find no cause.

"I think the borderline deficiencies are extremely common," Dr. Tkacz says. "It's what's called the 'tea and toast' syndrome. Older people living on Social Security or a pension find themselves short of money and don't eat as well as they should." Add to that teenagers subsisting on fast foods and people of any age who let life's stresses overtake their daily intake of B vitamins, and you've got quite a crowd.

"Some people have been brainwashed by traditional medicine into believing that we are getting all the nutrients we need in our average diet," says Dr. Picker. "But there are numerous large-scale studies to counter that fallacy. They show there is a large percentage of the American public that is below the Recommended Dietary Allowance (RDA) for many key nutrients, including some of the B vitamins."

So what's the best protection against a deficiency? Eating B-complex-rich foods is important. Organ meats like liver and kidneys are among the best sources. Just three ounces of beef liver contains more than 100 percent of the adult male RDA for riboflavin (vitamin B_2) and vitamin B_{12}, close to 100 percent for niacin and about 25 percent each for B_6 and folate. Whole grains, nuts, seeds and beans also contain good amounts. An alternative is B_{12}-fortified brewer's yeast or a good B-complex supplement.

"I have my patients take from one teaspoon to one tablespoon of brewer's yeast a day," Dr. Picker says. He also has them follow a diet that's high in fiber and complex carbohydrates, and low in fats and sweets. "I advise them to minimize or eliminate alcohol or caffeine intake, and I always give them a big lecture about smoking. All three of those are big users of the B vitamins."

"Just one simple step of providing B complex or brewer's yeast in the diet can eliminate a whole host of potential neurological and psychological problems," adds Dr. Tkacz.

The Best Meat You Can Eat

Beef's been on the grill for quite a few years now. "Eat less red meat," medical researchers have said, and we've listened. Fearful of cholesterol and fat, we've switched to more chicken and fish, and heaped our salad bowls high.

And—make no mistake—you *can* eat too much meat. A diet which serves up bacon, sausage, luncheon meats, steaks, chops, hamburgers or hot dogs several times a day is a diet almost certainly too high in fat and too low in fiber to be optimally healthful.

But there's another side to the meat story. If you choose the right cuts, prepare the meat properly, and eat it in moderation, meat can be positively health-building food.

Consider, first of all, this question. Which has more cholesterol: beef, chicken or fish? Almost everyone gets that one wrong. The answer is that they all have essentially the very same amount of cholesterol, about 75 milligrams or so to a four-ounce serving.

Second, the fat and calorie content of various cuts of beef and other meats varies from mammoth to surprisingly modest. Generalizations just don't work. Take a sirloin steak, for instance. Broil a six-ouncer as it comes out of a butcher's case and you've got 660 calories, including lots of fat. But trim away all the visible fat and you're left with a four-ounce steak that has only 350 calories. Fully 47 percent of the fat content has been eliminated.

Even more interesting, certain cuts of beef, such as round and flank steak, are quite lean to begin with. A broiled six-ounce round steak, untrimmed, has 440 calories. Cut away the ounce or so of fat on the steak, and you're down to 320 calories and a very respectable fat level.

Don't make the mistake, though, of cooking meat *with* its fat, and trimming it off at the table. Some of the fat that melts during cooking will actually be absorbed into the meat. So trim before cooking, then broil on a slatted tray that permits some of the remaining fat to drip away. The result is good, lean, nutritious eating.

And, of course, if you're cooking meat that's low in fat to begin with, you're better off yet. For details, see our list of various beef cuts and their percentage of calories from fat.

But what about *saturated* fat? Isn't beef higher in this kind of fat—believed to push cholesterol levels up—than chicken or fish? Generally, yes. But remember, generalizations can be deceiving. Choose the really lean cuts, like round, and ounce for ounce you've got a lot *less* saturated fat than we get from such common foods as stewed chicken, peanuts, cheese and even sunflower seeds.

On the plus side, beef is an extremely good source of protein, B vitamins, iron and zinc. The latter two minerals are believed to be deficient in many diets, particularly in those of women who are watching their weight.

And even a small amount of beef can greatly increase the amount of iron our bodies can absorb from grains, potatoes and vegetables. (Enter beef stew, stage right.)

However you cut it—or cook it—beef does have more fat than vegetables or fruits. But this is true of most protein-rich foods, including dairy products, nuts and seeds. The trick is to balance these foods with others that are extremely low in fat— fruits, vegetables, corn, rice, wheat and other grains, beans of all kinds, potatoes and pasta. Go easy on the butter and you wind up with a daily diet that excludes excess fat.

Many health authorities recommend a diet that derives no more than 30 percent of its total calories from fat. To see how that works in practice, let's begin with a well-trimmed porterhouse steak—not an especially lean piece of meat. About 42 percent of its calories come from fat. But if you include a four-ounce baked potato, one slice of whole wheat bread, four ounces of broccoli, one pat of butter and eight ounces of skim milk with your broiled steak (a four-ounce serving), you've reduced the ratio of calories from fat to 25 percent. The total calories from this typical dinner is a quite moderate 615.

Perhaps some comparisons with meatless dishes will help put beef's benefits in perspective:

● A macaroni-and-cheese dish, made with 1½ cups of ricotta, fontina and Cheddar cheeses, eight ounces of macaroni and 1 cup of milk, has about 45 percent of its calories tied up in fat. A flank steak, on the other hand, has only 34 percent of its calories in fat. In fact, most cuts of beef contain significantly less fat than comparable amounts of many cheeses (with Brie, Gouda, Cheddar, ricotta, Swiss and Romano among them).

● A quiche made with two cups of Cheddar, spinach, rice, three eggs and one cup of light cream has a staggering 74 percent of its calories coming from fat. No wonder real men don't touch the stuff.

Is 'Prime' Really Tops?

But short of taking a course in butcher-shop basics, what can a health-conscious consumer do to negotiate the meat morass? A good start would be to familiarize yourself with the meat industry's grading system. Its top rating is "prime," which means, according to the United States Department of Agriculture (USDA), that the meat is "the most tender, juicy and flavorful." What makes a prime cut flavorful and juicy is fat, not only the trimmable fat but also the marbling, the flecks of fat within the lean that are impossible to eliminate. If you purchase a prime cut, it's best to cut away the trimmable fat before cooking.

The meat industry's "choice" rating goes to cuts that don't quite have enough marbling to warrant the prime label. Still, these cuts are high in fat content and so should be carefully trimmed.

Ironically, as one moves down the meat industry's rating chart, one makes a healthful ascent. The "good" and "standard" ratings are given to cuts "which lack the juiciness and flavor of the higher grades," according to the USDA. The reason? There's less fat. So you have less waste, fewer calories and less cholesterol and, perhaps best of all, the healthier cuts cost less. Fortunately, the meat industry has been offering more of the leaner cuts in the market recently.

So your choices are many, as the accompanying table shows. Beef's gamut runs from the cuts of the loin portion, which should be consumed in moderation and in careful balance with other foods, to the cuts of the round portion of the steer, which fall within the government's 30 percent of calories from fat recommendation.

When you eat out, however, another problem arises: identifying the cuts. While most supermarkets use standard names for cuts of beef, restaurants use many aliases. And since there

RATING THE BEEF*

Cut	Calories	Fat (g.)	Percent-age of Calories from Fat
Eye round	214	7	29
Chuck steak	219	8	33
Sirloin	235	9	33
Flank steak	222	8	34
Rump	236	11	40
Porterhouse[1]	254	12	42
T-bone[2]	253	12	42
Ground beef[3]	248	13	47
Club steak	277	15	48
Rib eye[4]	273	15	50

*Figures are based on a 4-ounce serving, trimmed of visible fat, and cooked. Each cut provides about 35 grams of protein and about 4 miligrams of iron, as well as about 100 miligrams of cholesterol.

[1]Filet mignon and Chateaubriand can be included in this cut.
[2]Strip loin and New York strip are synonyms for this cut.
[3]10 percent fat by weight.
[4]Delmonico and Spencer steak are synonyms for this cut.

SOURCES: Adapted from
Nutritive Value of American Foods in Common Units, Agriculture Handbook No. 456, by Catherine F. Adams (Washington, D.C.: Agricultural Research Service, U.S. Department of Agriculture, 1975).
Composition of Foods, Agriculture Handbook No. 8, by Bernice K. Watt and Annabel L. Merrill (Washington, D.C.: Agricultural Research Service, U.S. Department of Agriculture, 1975).

is no beef-eater's thesaurus, you need a guide. A few of the more common noms de plume:

● Chateaubriand. This is a large tenderloin, sometimes called filet mignon. This is always at least a choice cut and it might be prime. It cost the restaurant more to get and it'll cost you more.

● Surf 'n' turf. You can ask the waiter wishfully if this is haddock and round steak, but typically this is a shellfish (usually lobster) and a tenderloin cut of beef that by itself would be filet mignon.

● London broil. This is a flank steak and a highly recommended cut at home or out. It'll cost you less in a market or a restaurant, and from a nutritional standpoint is one of the best cuts of beef.

Whether you're buying meat at the supermarket or ordering it at a restaurant, be assertive. Don't feel that you're inconveniencing the meat cutter by asking him to trim fat for you. And make it clear to the waiter that the size of his tip depends on whether or not you get the beef exactly the way you want it. This allows you to enjoy beef, not only without reservation but also with the knowledge that you're doing something good for yourself.

Zinc and Healing Update

It's been only 11 years since zinc was recognized as essential and given a Recommended Dietary Allowance (RDA) of 15 milligrams daily. But in that short time, this trace mineral has been shown to have a profound influence on the body's ability to grow and to resist disease. Male sexual maturity and fertility depend on adequate zinc. And some researchers think our declining ability to absorb zinc, along with other nutrients, as we age is one reason we become more vulnerable to disease.

So far, researchers have found more than 90 zinc-dependent

enzymes in the body—more than those of all the other minerals combined, including iron. Each is involved in a different biochemical reaction. But we need to know only two closely related facts about zinc to understand a good part of its importance.

First, zinc is needed for the body to make protein. Zinc-containing enzymes help to string together the long chains of amino acids that make up each molecule of protein.

Second, every cell's genetic material, its DNA and RNA, is derived from protein.

What this means is that your body needs zinc to make every one of its cells—from the hair on your head to the soles of your feet. Severe deficiencies mean that needed cells may not get made. They also mean that it is more difficult to repair damaged genetic material.

Because cell growth is so dependent on zinc, it's first missed when or where rapid cell growth occurs—in pregnancy, childhood, wound healing and any other situation involving rapidly dividing cells. One of these areas is the immune response.

"Severe zinc deficiency has been shown to cause major abnormalities in the body's immune defense," says Susanna Cunningham-Rundles, Ph.D., a researcher at Memorial Sloan-Kettering Cancer Center in New York City.

One reason for this impact is that any effective immune response involves a massive buildup of the white blood cells that fight bacteria, viruses and cancer. For instance, one type of white blood cell, called a neutrophil, can multiply five times within a few hours after infection sets in. And another kind of white blood cell, called a lymphocyte, can divide and form up to 500 new cells in four days.

"Studies show that if zinc is not present in the quantities needed, this sort of cell proliferation is reduced, and the immune response will be lessened," Dr. Cunningham-Rundles says.

And there are other roles zinc plays in the immune response.

"Zinc is probably essential for the work of thymic hormones," Dr. Cunningham-Rundles says. These hormones, secreted by the thymus gland, are responsible for development of T cells, types of lymphocytes central to the fight against viral and bacterial infections.

Zinc will also increase the activity of lymphocytes called

natural killer cells. Because these cells are able to destroy a virus-or bacteria-invaded cell without the prior sensitization that all other lymphocytes require, they are considered part of the body's first line of defense against disease.

Zinc also seems to interact with vitamin A, a nutrient that seems to have a protective effect against cancer.

Certain cells, called epithelial cells, may be particularly dependent on both A and zinc. These cells cover a surface, like the skin, or line a cavity, like the bladder. It's not incidental that these cells also have the most rapid turnover of any in the body. Or that throat cancers have been linked with deficiencies of both vitamin A and zinc.

Michael Bunk, Ph.D., a Memorial Sloan-Kettering research scientist, found that mice made zinc deficient also became deficient in vitamin A.

"It's pretty well shown that zinc deficiency affects the release of stored vitamin A from the liver," Dr. Bunk says. He thinks there may be a second connection, that a zinc deficiency impairs the uptake of vitamin A by the epithelial cells, putting them at risk for developing cancer or other diseases.

Links with Eating Disorders

Doctors have known for some time that too little zinc can alter the senses of taste and smell. A lack of zinc changes the chemistry of saliva, which directly affects the way things taste in the mouth. Zinc-poor people have trouble tasting sweets, for instance.

But zinc may also affect areas of the brain that receive and process information from taste and smell sensors. And that, in part, has led some researchers to speculate that zinc could influence areas of the brain that control eating and drinking behavior.

"Animal studies seem to indicate that zinc deficiencies could play a role in eating disorders like anorexia and bulimia," says Craig McClain, M.D., associate professor of medicine and director of the division of gastroenterology at the University of Kentucky School of Medicine, Lexington. Studies he and his colleagues have done indicate that zinc-deprived rats develop the same bizarre eating habits as teenage girls diagnosed as anorexic, bulimic or bulimirexic, a combination of both disorders. Like the girls, the zinc-deprived rats ate less and less, until they were consuming only about a third the normal amount. When they did eat, they tended to pig out, and they also tended to easily regurgitate their food. What's more, when they were subjected to stress (mildly pinched tails), they headed straight for the rat chow! When adequate zinc was added to their diet, the rats' eating behavior returned to normal (*Physiology and Behavior,* March, 1984).

In another study, Dr. McClain found that nine bulimirexic women were extremely low in zinc, even when they were within normal weight ranges and other nutritional signs were normal. "Many of these women's habits—laxative abuse, vomiting, dieting—would definitely put them at risk for a zinc deficiency," Dr. McClain says (*Clinical Research,* October, 1984).

One question is, which comes first, the zinc deficiency or the eating problem? "It's possible that a zinc-poor diet, which wouldn't be all that unusual in teenage girls, could trigger eating problems," Dr. McClain says. "Or the eating problem could be triggered by psychological or social problems."

Can zinc supplements help anorexics break the habit? Perhaps, Dr. McClain says. "That's what we intend to study next. Until results are in with humans, though, about the only recommendation I can give people with eating disorders is to make sure they're getting the RDA of zinc."

Zinc, Alcohol and Obesity

Surprising connections also seem to exist between zinc deficiencies, alcohol abuse and obesity, says Platon Collipp, M.D., professor of pediatrics at State University of New York, Stony Brook.

He found that rats fed zinc-deficient diets voluntarily drank much more alcohol than rats fed adequate zinc. (The rats could choose between water and alcohol in their cages.) When they were then given enough zinc, their drinking declined to normal (*Alcoholism: Clinical and Experimental Research,* November-December, 1984).

"People have been speculating for some time now that food intake can influence drinking behavior. I think zinc is one nutrient that could have a possible effect," says Dr. Collipp. "It would be very interesting to see how or if zinc reduces the craving for alcohol in alcoholics. I haven't been able to do that study, but it should be done. So should a study to see whether zinc supplementation in the children of alcoholics, who may be genetically zinc deficient, reduces their five-times-greater-than-normal chance of becoming alcoholics themselves."

Dr. Collipp also made an interesting discovery that may help some heavyweights. He found that a zinc deficiency is associated with the way the body handles glucose (blood sugar).

A zinc-dependent enzyme in the liver acts as a kind of railroad switch in glucose metabolism. Called a branch-point enzyme, it's located right at the spot in glucose metabolism where one reaction leads to energy burning and the other to fat storage.

"Studies of rat livers show that when there's not enough zinc to go around, this enzyme becomes inactive," Dr. Collipp says. "The result is that glucose is shunted toward making triglycerides (blood fats) that can be stored in the fatty tissues rather than being burned for energy" (*Pediatrics Annuals,* June, 1984).

"There are some people who say that everything they eat turns to fat," he says. "Well, those people may be zinc deficient."

A Satiation Link?

Dr. Collipp also thinks there may be psychological connections in zinc's effect on eating and drinking. Zinc-deficient children don't seem to rely on "internal cues" for their behavior, he says. Such children might not be able to discern the difference between feeling hungry and feeling full, for instance.

"Quite a few studies link zinc deficiencies with brain disorders, like learning problems," Dr. Collipp says. "I think a zinc deficiency may also affect some part of the brain involved in the self-monitoring of the body, a kind of satiation center that lets you know when you've had enough to eat or drink."

Healthy Gums Need Zinc

Zinc deficiency is especially detrimental to the gums. The tissue is loaded with fibrous protein strands, and the thin layers of cells right next to the tooth's root is epithelium, says Henry Mallek, D.M.D., Ph.D., professor at the Georgetown University School of Dentistry in Washington, D.C.

A zinc deficiency doesn't actually *cause* gum disease. Plaque does. But a deficiency makes the gums much less likely to be able to withstand the bacterial assault of plaque that inflames gums and loosens teeth.

"There are many reasons to think that people with gum disease may have zinc deficiencies," Dr. Mallek says. "I've seen people with long-term gum problems who had conventional treatment. Although it helped, the gums were not completely healthy. But when the zinc deficiency was corrected, the gum problems were resolved."

Zinc for Osteoporosis?

Osteoporosis is a hot topic these days. Increased calcium intake and weight-bearing exercises can help head it off. And it seems zinc might help, too.

Bone metabolism is another area where zinc-dependent enzymes play a role, says Joseph Soares, Ph.D., a professor of nutrition at the University of Maryland, College Park.

In bone calcification in children, the role is clear, Dr. Soares says. The zinc is needed to produce a matrix of protein threads onto which the bone-forming calcium is laid. In older people, though, the process is much slower. "Calcium deposition and removal continues into old age, but if more calcium is lost than is deposited, osteoporosis will be the result," Dr. Soares says.

"We'd like to find out if zinc can help to boost calcium deposition in the elderly. It would seem to make sense, but it's a difficult question to answer." Dr. Soares's current work will determine the role of supplementation in bone calcification in quail and rats. If it does, he says, "an important new development in the study and control of osteoporosis may be available."

A recent study by researchers in Turkey showed that victims of osteoporosis had zinc levels 25 percent lower than those without the disease. "Many older people are getting too little zinc, just as they're getting too little calcium, because of overall poor nutrition," Dr. Soares says. In fact, there's evidence to indicate that zinc intake is below the RDA for other groups as well.

A recent survey by the Beltsville Human Nutrition Research Center in Maryland found that middle-class adults were getting only about three-fourths of the RDA for zinc, averaging 9.9 milligrams a day. Women fared worst. Their intake was only 57 percent of the 15-milligram requirement. Based on these people's food choices, the researchers calculated it would take 3,000 calories a day for them to get the RDA of zinc!

Make your food choices zinc-wise. Three ounces of oysters, the richest source, has 143 milligrams of zinc. Meats are the next-best source. Three ounces of lean beef has 5.3 milligrams of zinc. Grains and nuts contain fairly good, but probably less absorbable, amounts. In fact, a nutritional survey showed vegetarians on low-calorie diets to be at particular risk for zinc deficiencies. (If you feel you need supplemental zinc, don't take more than 30 milligrams a day without medical supervision.)

Zinc research can only continue to confirm how important it is to get the right amount of this essential trace mineral.

Better Nutrition for Better Vision

The patient had cataracts. The normally transparent lenses of his eyes, which bring images down to their sharpest focus on the retina, had turned cloudier and cloudier until he was almost blind. The doctor operated on one eye to restore the patient's vision, and prescribed a multivitamin containing zinc. Then they waited for the eye to heal so the doctor could operate on the other eye. To their amazement, when the man returned to the doctor, the second cataract was gone. The patient ended up with 20/25 vision in both eyes—ten times better than when he first went in.

To Gary Price Todd, M.D., an ophthalmologist from Waynesville, North Carolina, and author of *Nutrition, Health and Disease* (Donning Book Co., 1985), that was the end of a diligent search and the beginning of a new way of practicing medicine. "In 1974, I was going through my ophthalmology residency at the National Naval Medical Center in Bethesda, Maryland. Part of my residency was a tour in Ethiopia with the International Eye Foundation. I found that the people in Ethiopia developed cataracts at a very young age—in their thirties and forties instead of their sixties and seventies, as is typical in the United States. I could find only one logical reason why they were developing cataracts so early. It had to be nutritional.

"The Ethiopians ate almost no vegetables, even though they were available then. They grew them and sold them to foreigners, but didn't eat them. Two Ethiopian women cooked for us while we were there, and they were surprised that anyone could eat so many vegetables—their diet wasn't as varied. Most of the time they ate a stew consisting of a peppery sauce on thin bread. It was obvious that their diet was inadequate.

"My experience in Ethiopia convinced me that cataracts could be of nutritional origin. And if *they* were developing cataracts for nutritional reasons, *we* probably were also. It's just that our diet was enough better than it stalled things off for a couple of decades.

"From then on I started looking for the nutritional factors that might reverse cataracts. I gave my patients multivitamins, but to no avail. Then in 1979, I tried a new multivitamin product on the market that contained zinc, and it worked. The man's cataract disappeared. At that point I figured zinc was the key.

"The same day the man came back with good vision, a woman came in with cataracts and 20/60 vision in each eye. A person with 20/60 vision can't pass a driver's exam and can't read without magnification. Instead of scheduling surgery, I put her on the same zinc-containing multivitamin and brought her back six weeks later to see what had happened. Her vision had improved to 20/30 in each eye. Six weeks after that she was 20/20 in each eye, where she remains to this day. At that point I stopped doing surgery until every one of my patients had a reasonable chance to see if the supplement would work."

There is some scientific evidence to back up Dr. Todd's experience. When researchers at a United States Department of the Interior laboratory fed trout either a low-zinc diet or the same diet with a zinc supplement, 75 percent of the trout on the zinc-poor diet developed cataracts. None of the trout on the zinc-supplemented diet developed cataracts (*Federation Proceedings,* March 1, 1978). In addition, doctors have reported cataracts in children with acrodermatitis enteropathica, a zinc-deficiency disease (*Skin and Allergy News,* October, 1979).

However, not all of Dr. Todd's cataract patients responded to zinc. So when he later read that B-vitamin deficiency can cause cataracts, he added them to his anticataract arsenal. But a few patients still did not respond. Then he made an unusual discovery. While treating patients with vitamin E for other eye problems, he found that their cataracts also cleared. It wasn't until later, though, that he found out why.

Shedding Light on Cataracts

Current research supports the theory that cataracts can be caused by an excess of free radicals in the lens of the eye. Free radicals are highly reactive chemicals that are generated by a normal chemical process in the body called oxidation. Left unchecked, free radicals can initiate reactions that result in unwanted tissue changes. Because light also promotes oxidation, the transparent tissues of the eye are particularly susceptible to free-radical damage.

Shambhu D. Varma, Ph.D., of the department of ophthalmology at the University of Maryland Medical School, is investigating the role of free radicals in cataract formation, and cataract prevention by antioxidant nutrients. In test-tube experiments, Dr. Varma maintained rat lenses in a fluid that generates free radicals when exposed to light. He found that the lenses lost their transparency. "Oxidation is one of the factors contributing to the pathogenesis of cataracts," says Dr. Varma, "although there might be other causes, too."

Because it's an antioxidant, Dr. Varma and his colleagues wanted to see if vitamin C would have a beneficial effect. Again, rat lenses were maintained in a special mixture that caused free-radical damage. But lenses maintained in the same mixture fortified with vitamin C were significantly protected from damage by free radicals. According to the researchers, that may explain why there is such a high level of vitamin C in the eye (*Proceedings of the National Academy of Sciences,* July, 1979). In a similar study, Dr. Varma and his co-workers found that vitamin E also offered protection against cataracts (*Photochemistry and Photobiology,* vol. 36, no. 6, 1982).

"I recently did a study with a strain of mice that have a tendency to develop cataracts. I found they don't develop them as much as expected if they're given vitamin E," Dr. Varma reports. "A good diet is established to be necessary for the maintenance of a healthy, transparent, pliable lens. If your diet is deficient in antioxidant vitamins E and C, chances of developing cataracts might be accelerated," he says.

When Dr. Todd became aware of the role of free radicals in cataract formation, he added antioxidant vitamins and minerals to the supplements he was already prescribing for his cataract patients. The full regimen includes 500 milligrams of vitamin C, 400 international units (I.U.) of vitamin E, 200 micrograms of selenium, 20 milligrams of zinc and 20 milligrams of manganese, along with extra amounts of B-complex vitamins. "If a patient is deficient in zinc and develops a cataract because of that, zinc will reverse it to a degree. But if the deficiency isn't zinc but selenium, then the zinc isn't going to do him a whole lot of good. What it's coming down to," claims Dr. Todd, "is that there's a chain of biochemical events and every link has to be there in adequate quantities to neutralize free radicals."

Retina Also Affected

The retina, the membrane at the back of the eye that receives the image formed by the lens, may also be susceptible to free-radical damage. After seven years of ongoing study, Ely J. Crary, M.D., of Smyrna, Georgia, says he's found a way to retard the progression of diabetic retinopathy, a disease of the retina that frequently leads to blindness. He uses a combination of the antioxidants selenium and vitamins E, C and A.

He theorizes that in diabetics, decreased metabolism in the cells of the eye's blood vessels is caused by a buildup of free radicals, or oxidants. This weakens the capillary cell walls, leading to blood leakage. It's this vascular leakage that's responsible for the early loss of sight. Antioxidants remove the oxidants, preventing further damage.

"I've worked with close to 1,000 patients with diabetic retinopathy and senile macular degeneration," Dr. Crary declares, "and have seen the diseases retarded in about 70 percent of the cases. This program of nutritional supplementation has shown no adverse effects, either. If someone has early diabetic retinopathy or senile macular degeneration, they should at least consider this program in addition to regular therapy— under a doctor's care, of course. The earlier the treatment is started, the better the response. I'm still amazed at the results we get from this method."

Dr. Todd has also had good results with both diabetic retinopathy and senile macular degeneration. "In 1981, a woman came in with 20/60 vision in each eye due to senile macular degeneration. At this point it's the physician's unhappy duty to inform the patient that they have a disease that's likely to be progressive and destroy their ability to read even very large print, and that there's nothing the physician can do about it. The central portion of the retina starts deteriorating and gradually ceases to function. The central one millimeter of the retina is the only part that sees 20/20. The rest of the retina sees about 20/400 at best. Senile macular degeneration is today the number one cause of incurable blindness.

"I told her the brutal facts of the disease and said 'there's a possibility that vitamin E might help you.' In approximately three months her vision came from 20/60 to 20/30," Dr. Todd says. "After six months her vision was 20/20, and it still is. Since then, I've treated almost 30 patients with macular degeneration in this manner. Over 90 percent have had their vision partially or completely restored, including two patients whose vision had deteriorated to the point where they could barely see my hand move in front of them. In those severe cases it was almost a year before we saw any improvement.

"What I tell my patients today is, 'We'll wait one year to see if treatment is effective. Don't give up hope. I've seen people almost totally blind whose vision was restored to the point where they could pass their driver's exam,'" he continues.

Many research studies have tied vitamin E to the health of

the retina. In a study at Cornell University, dogs fed diets deficient in vitamin E were found to develop damaged retinas. Damage could be detected after only three months on the E-deficient diet. "Night blindness and eventual severe day visual impairment" followed, say the researchers (*American Journal of Veterinary Research,* January, 1981).

Retrolental fibroplasia (RLF) is a disease of the retina in premature infants that causes blindness. In the 1950s, it was discovered that oxygen therapy in incubators was the cause, and careful monitoring of oxygen levels caused a decline in the incidence of severe RLF. However, there was a resurgence of the disease as more very small premature infants were able to survive.

Recently, researchers from the department of newborn medicine at the Royal Alexandra Hospital in Edmonton, Alberta, found that vitamin E can prevent RLF in infants given oxygen. In the study, 17 percent of the tiny infants who received no vitamin E developed RLF, while none of the infants given oral vitamin E within 12 hours of birth developed RLF. Say the researchers, "It is recommended that vitamin E be given within 12 hours of birth to all [low-birth-weight] infants . . . who require supplemental oxygen" (*Ophthalmology,* vol. 90, no. 5, 1983).

Reducing Eye Pressure

Chronic glaucoma is another eye disease that Dr. Todd treats with nutritional along with conventional therapy. "In glaucoma, the drainage holes in the eye clog up and the fluid doesn't drain properly. Pressure inside the eye builds. It restricts blood flow in the eye and the flow of nutrients inside the nerve cells. It's like when you sit with your legs crossed and your foot goes to sleep. In this case, the optic nerve goes to sleep. Vision is lost slowly over a period of years, so slowly that the patient rarely notices. He is totally unaware of the loss of vision until he is nearly blind. That's why regular examinations by an ophthalmologist are important." Glaucoma is responsible for almost 50 percent of all cases of adult blindness, and strikes more than 2 percent of those over 40 years of age.

"Traditional medicines aren't effective for all patients. They're about 80 to 90 percent effective. And if the pressure doesn't come down, surgery is the next step. The type of surgery done depends on the type of glaucoma. In many cases laser surgery can be effective," says Dr. Todd.

"If someone comes in with glaucoma, I start treating them with traditional medicines along with vitamin A and manganese to reduce the pressure. About six months later, I begin reducing the medication. About 40 percent of the patients are able to stop taking the medication and stay just on the vitamins.

"On electron microscope scanning you can see abnormal mucopolysaccharides blocking the drainage sites in the eye of those people with glaucoma. Vitamin A and manganese are both important for proper mucopolysaccharide synthesis. In 1982 I did 22 glaucoma operations, in 1983 I did 3, and last year only 1 patient needed glaucoma surgery. Yet my glaucoma practice today is larger than ever before. Nutritional treatment does work, but it's probably more effective to maintain good nutrition throughout life than try to reverse damage once it's done," Dr. Todd advises.

World Report on Vitamins against Cancer

The old theory that certain vitamins may have anticancer powers is dead, replaced by a new reality that's slowly being refined and tested by scientists from around the world. Can nutrients magnify the positive effects of chemotherapy or radiation? Can vitamins attack a malignant tumor or prevent one from occurring? Can they increase the life expectancy of some terminal cancer patients? All the evidence on these questions isn't in yet, but the existing data are far more encouraging than most people realize.

"With various nutrients, we have for the first time in human history a biological tool to prevent cancer," says Kedar N. Prasad, Ph.D., a researcher at the University of Colorado Health Sciences Center and president of the International Association for Vitamins and Nutritional Oncology. "And the prospects for treatment with nutrients look promising as well.

It will take a long time before we have conclusive evidence of all the anticancer properties of these substances, but we've made a good start."

Most researchers in the field would probably agree, and most of the latest scientific news on the subject bears them out. Here's a sampling of studies (most of them so recent they're unpublished) that helps define the status of vitamins in the cancer wars.

Fukuoka, Japan

Noted scientist Fukumi Morishige, M.D., Ph.D., and his colleagues report more progress in their treatment of seriously ill cancer patients with vitamin C.

For 30 years Dr. Morishige has been examining the healing potential of vitamin C. Seven years ago he published data suggesting that large doses of the nutrient may increase the survival times of terminal cancer patients, and since then he and his fellow researchers have been successfully treating cancer patients with combinations of C and other therapies. The latest news is that they may have just discovered how to make vitamin C more of a tumor killer than most researchers ever imagined.

Through a series of test-tube and animal studies, they found out that a mixture of C and a copper compound has surprisingly lethal effects on cancers—more lethal than either substance alone. When they treated cancerous mice with this mixture, the animals' life spans increased. And when they used it to treat a woman with terminal cancer, the results were astounding.

She was 34 years old and the victim of osteosarcoma, an incurable bone cancer completely resistant to chemotherapy. A tumor in her left arm was causing paralysis and so much pain that painkillers were worthless. Then she was injected regularly with the copper compound and large doses of vitamin C.

"Two months' treatment relieved the intolerable pain and paresis [paralysis] of the diseased left upper arm," Dr. Marishige reports. "From x-ray examinations the tumor lesion was found to be completely regressed [disappeared] and calcified within four months of treatment." Almost two years later the woman was still free of cancer.

Pavia, Italy

Leonida Santamaria, M.D., and his colleagues at the University of Pavia have uncovered preliminary evidence suggesting that beta-carotene (a precursor of vitamin A) may actually inhibit skin cancer.

The researchers conducted a study to see if beta-carotene—shown in a score of studies to have possible anticancer properties—could prevent skin cancer in mice exposed to a carcinogen and ultraviolet rays, the cancer-causing component of ordinary sunlight. The results revealed that exposed mice fed beta-carotene developed far less skin cancer than those not supplemented with the nutrient.

This study and the researchers' other experiments have convinced them that beta-carotene has an antitumor effect because it's an antioxidant—it helps the body thwart the cancer-causing process known as oxidation, a chemical chain reaction that can be triggered by several factors, including ultraviolet light.

"Our data," says Dr. Santamaria, "suggest the possibility that beta-carotene could be used to actually deter skin cancer in humans. And one advantage of such a use is that beta-carotene is absolutely nontoxic."

Los Angeles, California

Researchers from UCLA School of Medicine and Harbor-UCLA Medical Center have discovered that, at least in the laboratory, vitamin K may be as tough on tumors as chemotherapy or radiation.

They first removed a variety of malignant tumors from patients —from the breast, colon, ovary, lung and other places—then under special laboratory conditions subjected the tumors to vitamin K. And instead of continuing to grow, most of the tumors were stopped cold.

"These cancer-inhibiting effects," says chief researcher Rowan T. Chlebowski, M.D., Ph.D., "are comparable to those we would get with conventional cancer therapies."

Vitamin K's potency, however, wasn't exactly a surprise to Dr. Chlebowski and his team. Other investigators had previously demonstrated that giving certain cancer patients vitamin K along with standard radiation treatments could help the patients live longer.

"Our next step," Dr. Chlebowski told us, "is to find out what vitamin K alone can do to tumors when we administer it directly to patients."

Denver, Colorado

Investigators at the University of Colorado Health Sciences Center have discovered in laboratory tests that vitamin E may halt the growth of prostate-cancer cells.

Test-tube research had already shown that E could kill or inhibit other kinds of malignant cells, but this study is the first word on vitamin E's impact on cancer of the prostate.

"Our data suggest," says Dr. Prasad, one of the researchers in the study, "that vitamin E may be useful in the treatment of patients with prostatic cancer. After all, compared to cancer drugs, vitamin E is very low in toxicity, so it can be easily incorporated into chemotherapy treatments. It simply will not interfere with standard therapy."

Philadelphia, Pennsylvania

Using 13-cis retinoic acid (a derivative of vitamin A), scientists at the Medical College of Pennsyvlania have treated patients and achieved startling results—some of the patients actually went into remission.

The researchers gave 13-cis retinoic acid to 18 people with myelodysplastic syndrome (MDS), a preleukemia disease that responds only sporadically to chemotherapy, rarely goes into remission, and is invariably fatal. After several months of this therapy, two of the people went into partial remission for two to five months, and two went into complete remission for up to two years.

"These long complete remissions are remarkable," says head researcher Emanuel C. Besa, M.D. "I know of no chemotherapy that has ever produced such lengthy remissions in this disease. And you have to remember that when we treat MDS with chemotherapy, normal cells are wiped out along with the malignant ones. The advantage of 13-cis retonoic acid is that it can effect remission without such side effects.

"Obviously, not all MDS patients respond to 13-cis, but a subgroup of them will. We find this very encouraging," he says.

And so is much of the news from the front—the news of the role of vitamins in the cancer wars.

PUTTING ANTICANCER VITAMINS IN YOUR DIET

Does the recent research linking cancer and nutritional factors suggest a dietary game plan for preventing cancer?

Many scientists say yes, and offer dietary recommendations for reducing cancer risk. Among the suggestions are:

• Eat fruits and vegetables daily, especially those high in vitamin C and beta-carotene (like grapefruit, oranges, mangoes, cabbage, spinach, carrots, turnip greens and sweet potatoes).
• Eat foods high in fiber, such as whole grain cereals, peas, lentils, sweet corn, potatoes, parsnips, pears and strawberries.
• Eat fewer foods high in saturated fats, such as deep-fried dishes and fatty cuts of meat.

How Much Coffee Can *You* Handle?

Although in recent years some scientists have considered the rich, dark brew to be simmering with potential health hazards, coffee is enjoying some revisionist thinking these days. It may not be as bad as you once thought—provided, of course, you practice moderation. In fact, you might be the best judge of how "good" coffee is for you and how much is too much.

The source of controversy over coffee is its most studied (though not necessarily largest) constituent, caffeine. Generally considered to be the most widely used drug in America and Europe, caffeine is an often powerful central nervous system stimulant that, in some people, can cause modest increases in blood pressure and heart rate, arrhythmias, anxiety and sleeplessness.

For most people, caffeine taken in modest amounts is a pretty harmless and pleasurable vice. "If you're a normal person, your body can cope with 300 milligrams of caffeine a day—that's about three cups of coffee," says Manfred Kroger, Ph.D., professor of food science at Pennsylvania State University and a spokesman for the Institute of Food Technologists.

He cautions, however, that coffee, which contains literally hundreds of less studied chemicals in addition to caffeine, can be ambrosia to one and hemlock to another. Response to a cup of java can be as individual as fingerprints.

"I, for instance, am not a 'normal' person," says Dr. Kroger. "If I drink three cups of coffee in the afternoon, I'll be up until midnight. If I drink one cup after 6:00, I'll be up until 3:00. I haven't given up coffee entirely. I've learned to work around my sensitivity."

Most people do. Coffee has a way of tipping off the body when enough is enough. "It seems that if you take too much you tend not to take any more," says Peter Dews, M.D., Ph.D., professor of psychiatry and psychobiology at Harvard Medical School and editor of *Caffeine, Perspectives from Recent Research* (Springer-Verlag, 1984). "Suppose, for instance, you drink coffee during a business meeting. If you start feeling uncomfortable, you stop. That's why you see so many half-drunk cups of coffee lying around after meetings in a way you rarely see half-drunk cups of soft drinks. At a subliminal level, there's an automatic stop with coffee. You don't even have to think about it."

But a lot of people are thinking about their coffee drinking—and worrying about it, since some research studies have linked coffee drinking to heart disease, cancer and even birth defects. So, here are a few answers to the most troubling questions you may have about the last of your "vices."

Will Coffee Make Me Nervous and Irritable?

It can. The most common side effects of coffee are nervousness and insomnia, and whether you experience them depends largely on how much caffeine you're getting and your individual susceptibility. You'll have to let your past coffee experiences be your guide.

"Your body will tell you," says Dr. Kroger. "People should learn to observe their bodies the way they do their cars."

Your body, like your car, can have its knocks and pings. You may be drinking too much if you're unusually nervous, restless or battling with insomnia—that's the old coffee jitters. You could also be overdosing if you're experiencing heart palpitations, diarrhea, headache or heartburn. In some people, coffee acts as a diuretic, so you may have increased urine output.

Quantitatively, excessive consumption can be considered anything over four cups of strongly brewed coffee a day, which can lead to what doctors call caffeinism. The symptoms are identical to—and are sometimes mistaken for—anxiety neurosis. Caffeinism affects as many as one in ten people.

How caffeine affects you personally may depend on your own metabolism or whether you drink coffee on a regular basis. One of the problems researchers face when studying the effects of caffeine on humans is that it affects habitual consumers and nonconsumers quite differently, say Peter Curatolo, M.D., and David Robertson, M.D., who reviewed the myriad caffeine studies for *Annals of Internal Medicine* (vol. 96, no. 5, 1983).

For instance, when a group of nondrinkers was given a daily dose of 250 milligrams of caffeine (equivalent to about 2½ cups of coffee), these so-called caffeine-naive people experienced small increases in blood pressure, heart rate and excretion of stress hormones from the adrenal gland. So did a group of habitual drinkers—who had abstained for three weeks before the test—when they were given 250 milligrams of caffeine three times a day for a week. The difference, however, was that the habitual drinkers developed a tolerance to the caffeine long before the week was up and no longer had any untoward reactions.

Will Coffee Keep Me Up at Night?

Your metabolism—specifically, how quickly your system eliminates caffeine—may determine whether coffee keeps you up at night. In a study at Jerusalem's Hadassah University Hospital, researchers found that people who said coffee kept them up consumed less coffee—explained by their bad reaction to it—and eliminated it more slowly from their systems than people who claimed coffee didn't affect their sleep.

The researchers concluded that individual metabolism dictates whether coffee will rob you of a good night's sleep or not bother you at all.

Why Do I Drink Coffee?

It may be because of the taste or because of the nice buzz it gives you, making you feel that "God's in his heaven and all's right with the world." In a Swiss study, volunteers who drank the equivalent of one cup of coffee said they felt full of ideas and go, with greater vigor, alertness and energy. Other researchers have found that caffeine can increase reading speed without increasing errors, improve the capacity for sustained intellectual effort and lead to less aggressive behaviors. There is even some indication that coffee increases aerobic capacity, which can give an athlete more staying power.

But be forewarned: What coffee gives, coffee may take away. Some people experience a poststimulation letdown that can make them as tired and lethargic as they were alert and energetic. One problem you can face if you treat coffee as more than simply a satisfying beverage is that you'll start to reach for more than you can handle just to prolong the kick.

Coffee can be mildly addicting. Any coffee drinker who's given it up cold turkey can tell you about the caffeine withdrawal headache and the bouts of weariness and lethargy, which, though quite real, aren't dangerous or permanent. Says Dr. Dews, "Caffeine addiction isn't an addiction in the traditional sense. It's part of your lifestyle. You become attached to that cup in the morning and you miss it when you don't have it. People are that way about orange juice. They can't even talk without their orange juice. But coffee isn't as hard to give up as cigarettes, and you're not likely to drive 30 miles in the snow for a cup of coffee."

Are There Any Long-Term Health Effects from Drinking Coffee?

Early studies linked caffeine with heart disease and cancer, but since then most of those findings have been disputed and most medical experts believe there's no clear evidence supporting them. But moderation is the key. The most recent study on coffee's role in heart disease, done at Stanford University, found that sedentary men between 30 and 55 who drink three cups or more of coffee a day may be at higher risk of developing heart disease than those who drink less coffee.

There is some indication that heavy coffee consumption, when accompanied by other diet and lifestyle factors, may increase cholesterol levels, a finding of several previous studies done outside the United States. There was no such association found when the men limited their coffee to two cups or fewer a day (*Journal of the American Medical Association,* March 8, 1985).

Are There Any Special Health Problems Coffee May Aggravate?

Coffee probably ought to be taken off the menu of people with ulcers or those who have experienced heartburn or other gastrointestinal problems, such as esophageal reflux, after drinking coffee. Coffee seems to promote gastric acid secretion. People with hypertension or heart disease who experience an increase in blood pressure or heart arrhythmias when drinking coffee should follow their common sense and switch to decaffeinated coffee or a less stimulating beverage. Coffee can cause modest increases in blood pressure and heart rate and, in large amounts—more than nine cups a day—is associated with arrhythmia.

Other people who ought to exercise caution are those with anemia (coffee inhibits the absorption of iron) and people who experience panic attacks, such as agoraphobics. Researchers at Yale University recently found that caffeine produces a more pronounced reaction in people who have panic episodes than in normal, healthy people.

There are also a number of studies that indicate a link between coffee and tea drinking and fibrocystic breast disease, a condition characterized by benign breast lumps. Other findings, however, have cast doubts on the association. The jury is still out, but some doctors advise women with the condition to avoid caffeinic beverages.

How Does Coffee Affect My Nutrition?

There's some evidence that coffee can inhibit the absorption of both iron and the B vitamin thiamine. In the case of thiamine, it doesn't appear to be caffeine that's the culprit but another coffee chemical, chlorogenic acid, which isn't shed during the decaffeinating process.

How Can I Enjoy Coffee without Worrying?

Although moderation is the key to coffee comfort, for some the most logical step is to switch to decaffeinated coffee. Many people can't tell the difference between "decaf" and the real thing. But if you can, you might want to stick to either instant or percolated coffee which, depending on how strong you make it, can contain less caffeine on average than drip coffee.

Adding milk to coffee won't cut down on caffeine, although it tends to slow its absorption. But café au lait, that delicious French way of serving coffee by filling half the cup with hot milk and half with dark coffee, will reduce the caffeine by reducing the amount of coffee in your cup. Substitute skim or low-fat milk and you eliminate calories and cholesterol as well.

Folate for Healthier Babies

When Miriam L., a coal miner's wife in the village of Gwent, Wales, gave birth to a healthy girl, she experienced all the joy and relief that a woman feels at the end of a successful pregnancy, and then some. Her previous child had been born with spina bifida, a crippling neural tube defect (NTD), and the 5 percent risk of having another handicapped child had hovered over her second pregnancy like a malignant cloud.

The two deliveries couldn't have been less alike, and yet the difference between them may have been nothing more than a few hundred micrograms a day of a B vitamin called folate. Miriam had taken part in a study conducted by Welsh researchers, who asked her and more than 100 women like herself to eat a good diet including high-folate foods before and during their next pregnancies. Like her, every woman who followed the researchers' advice later gave birth to a healthy baby.

Seldom has so little gone so far, and these results seemed to support something that's long been suspected: Folate (or folic acid) is the single most important nutrient for pregnant women and their developing children. In fact, eating fresh fruit and vegetables (which are rich in folate) from conception until the due date might be the best policy a woman can adopt to ensure that her pregnancy will be a happy and a healthy one.

Why folate? Because, on the cellular level, folate is a kind of molecular "midwife." It is one of the catalysts that helps bring new cells into this world. It is a key element in an enzyme that makes possible the duplication of DNA, which, in turn, enables one cell to split into two, then two into four, and so on. Without folate, growth simply slows down. Or it may be distorted and produce birth defects.

Besides NTDs, cleft palate and low birth weight or even miscarriage can come of a low-folate pregnancy. Aside from that, a woman may develop anemia or an inflammation of the gums called gingivitis as a result of the infant's demands on her folate supply. When it comes to folate, a pregnant woman is truly eating for two, and the National Academy of Sciences has decreed that pregnant women need twice as much folate a day as other adults.

Preventing Neural Tube Defects

It was to find out whether or not folate could prevent a second NTD delivery that the investigators, headed by Dr. K. M. Laurence, of the Welsh National School of Medicine, chose to study several hundred women in Wales. These women had, for the most part, delivered children with spina bifida or anencephaly, two potentially crippling or fatal NTDs in which the spine or skull fails to form around the spinal cord or brain. On the average, 15 out of every 10,000 women in the United States deliver NTD babies. But in this group, because of their history, the risk was 1 in 20.

Dr. Laurence and his assistants made a two-part study of these women. First they took a survey and discovered that fully half of them had had a poor diet during the pregnancy that ended with an NTD birth. Then they counseled 103 women to improve their diets in time for their next pregnancies. An additional 71 women were given no special dietary counseling.

Of the women who did improve their diets, none delivered a second handicapped child. All eight of the NTD children (out of 186 newborns) were born to women who ate a poor diet during the first six months of pregnancy (*Nutrition and Health,* vol. 2, no. 3/4, 1983).

"It seems likely that the main cause, in the British Isles at least, is a lack of folate available to the developing embryo," says Dr. Laurence, adding that the results of earlier work by himself and others "suggest that folic acid given to high-risk women greatly reduces the [NTD] recurrence rate," when taken before conception and continued until the end of the first trimester. Although Dr. Laurence concludes that some of the women in this latest study obtained enough folate from their diet alone to prevent a second NTD birth, he previously used a supplement of four milligrams a day—much more than would be available in the usual daily diet—for women at high risk for an NTD baby.

A Broader Role for Folate

Cleft palate, another birth abnormality, may also yield to a high-folate diet. Cleft palate occurs when an unborn child's facial bones fail to form properly, creating a distorting split in the roof of the mouth. Though not as traumatic as NTD, cleft palate can be socially crippling.

On hearing about the results of the English NTD studies, doctors in Czechoslovakia asked over 80 women who had already had a child with cleft palate to take ten milligrams of folate a day, along with a multivitamin, for at least three months before conception and then until at least the end of their first trimester. In 85 pregnancies, only one child was born with a cleft palate. In 212 pregnancies among a similar group where there was no supplementation, 15 cleft palates occurred. (*Lancet,* July, 1982).

There are even references in the medical literature linking low folate in a mother's diet to unwanted abortion and to low birth weight. As long ago as 1977, British researchers found that mothers with low folate levels at the time of delivery were more likely to deliver low-birth-weight children (*Archives of Disease in Childhood,* January, 1977).

As for spontaneous abortion, Carl C. Pfeiffer, M.D., Ph.D., of the Brain Bio Center in Princeton, New Jersey, writes that, "Many women with histories of abortion and miscarriage have been able to complete successful childbirth subsequent to folate supplementation" (*International Journal of Environmental Studies,* vol. 17, 1981).

Fragile-X: Handle with Folate

Sometimes folate can help repair the effects of birth defects after they occur—perhaps even long after they occur. Recently, folate supplements have been used to improve the mental function and the quality of life among mentally retarded children who suffer from what is called fragile-X syndrome. This syndrome, which appears under the microscope as a breakage in certain chromosomes, affects about 1 in every 1,000 newborns. In some cases, folate—if given early enough and in the right amounts—can raise the IQs of these children. In borderline cases, it might enable them to return to the mainstream of life.

Much work in this area has been done at the Children's Hospital Child Development Unit in Denver. A clinical researcher there, Tad Jackson, and Randi Hagerman, M.D., gave ten milligrams of folate a day to a group of boys with fragile-X syndrome. In the most remarkable case, one boy's IQ rose from 63 to a near-normal 86, then fell to 83 after folate was withdrawn. When the supplement was reintroduced, his IQ stabilized at 93.

"It's not a cure," says Jackson, "but in most cases folate

seems to improve the interaction between these children and the world around them. They talk more, they make better eye contact.

"The most encouraging sign has been that the parents of seven out of the eight boys under age 12 could tell by their behavior when their sons were taking folate, or not. In the boys over 12, however, not much improvement was seen."

Requirements Rise with Pregnancy

How much folate does a pregnant woman need? The National Academy of Sciences sets the Recommended Dietary Allowance (RDA) of folate for expectant mothers at 800 micrograms (0.8 milligram) a day and at 400 micrograms for other adults. These figures are low compared to the 4 milligrams some studies have suggested for NTD mothers.

In fact, the U.S. Food and Drug Administration (USDA) cautiously limits the potency of folate supplements sold in the United States to a maximum of 400 micrograms per tablet. The reason for the caution isn't because folate itself is hazardous. It is because folate taken in even normal amounts can mask the symptoms of megaloblastic anemia, which is an early sign of vitamin B_{12} deficiency. Testing their patients for vitamin B_{12} deficiency before prescribing greater-than-RDA doses of folate is one way that doctors avoid this problem.

Certain drugs can deprive us of folate and increase our need. Drugs for epilepsy, such as Dilantin, as well as barbiturates and methotrexate, an antipsoriasis drug, have this effect. Oral contraceptives, estrogen and alcohol are also known to reduce body folate levels.

Keep in mind, too, that the folate in foods can easily be reduced during cooking or processing. Heating foods or merely storing them at room temperature can cut their folate content in half. And beware of the folate vicious circle. A folate deficiency can actually make it more difficult for the walls of the intestines to absorb the folate it badly needs. Supplementation can break this cycle.

You may already be getting the folate you need from your diet, however. If fresh vegetables, especially spinach, romaine and asparagus, are a part of your diet, you are halfway there.

Lentils and dried beans, two foods that are high in fiber, also contain large amounts of folate. So do brewer's yeast, whole wheat bread and orange juice.

U.S. Study Planned

What does the future hold for the use of folate in the prevention of birth defects? Broader knowledge of the importance of folate in a pregnant woman's diet is necessary if the NTD occurrence rate is to come down, Dr. Laurence says.

Certain questions are still open. Should women who have *not* had a child with an NTD take folate supplements to prevent a first one? The vast majority—more than 90 percent—of NTD births fall in this category. Can a woman tell if she is at risk? Should all women of childbearing age take extra folate? Until answers are found, researchers call for better education about the problem.

"To reduce substantially the number of NTDs in the community, one must aim to improve the maternal diet through health education, which should be an integral and important part of the school curriculum," the Welsh researcher says. He sees a definite need for such a nutritional approach "in the immediate future."

Meanwhile, the U.S. Centers for Disease Control (CDC) in Atlanta are looking into this issue. The CDC and the Spina Bifida Association of America are considering launching a long-term study on the effects of folate supplements on women who have had NTD babies.

Over the next five years, researchers will give either a folate or nonfolate supplement to 350 female volunteers to find out if those taking supplements have fewer NTD recurrences.

The outlook so far? "At this point, we're not ready to recommend folate supplements to all women," CDC's M. J. Adams, M.D., told us recently. "We can't say for sure whether they are helpful or harmful. Some women may need more or less than others. But it's an exciting hypothesis, and I think women who are at risk for an NTD should become familiar with the uses of folate and other vitamin supplements before their next pregnancy."

FOOD SOURCES OF FOLATE

Food	Portion	Folate (mcg.)
Brewer's yeast	1 tablespoon	313
Tempeh, raw	3½ ounces	156
Broccoli, cooked	1 medium stalk	123
Liver, cooked	3 ounces	123
Spinach, raw	1 cup	109
Romaine, raw	1 cup	76
Black-eyed peas, cooked	½ cup	66
Asparagus, cooked	4 medium spears	59
Brussels sprouts, cooked	4 sprouts	50
Tomato juice	1 cup	48
Beets, cooked	½ cup	45
Orange juice	1 cup	45
Parsnips, cooked	½ cup	45
Lentils, raw	½ cup	38
Wheat germ, toasted	1 tablespoon	30
Collards, raw	1 cup	21
Kale, cooked	1 cup	17
Whole wheat bread	1 slice	10
Onions, raw	¼ cup	8

SOURCES: Adapted from
Composition of Foods: Vegetables and Vegetable Products, Agriculture Handbook No. 8-11, by Nutrition Monitoring Division (Washington, D.C.: Human Nutrition Information Service, U.S. Department of Agriculture, 1984. USDA Nutrition Data Research Branch.

Lifestyles That Crimp Nutrition

Quick! What are the four basic food groups? What does romaine lettuce have that iceberg doesn't? How about brown rice over white? What foods are rich in magnesium? Potassium? Zinc? What's a healthy amount of fat to have in your diet? How about protein? Fiber? And—take a guess—just how many "essential nutrients" are there, anyway? (Hint: You *won't* find the answer by counting the ingredients on a multivitamin bottle label.)

If you answered even the first question correctly (see the end of this chapter for answers), you're ahead of the crowd, some nutritionists say. And if you got every one right, you're excused from class. You really know the details when it comes to nutrition, and if you use that knowledge to eat better, you can count yourself one of the lucky few.

Research shows many Americans are increasingly concerned about what's in the 1,500 pounds of food they chow down each year. They're eating fewer frankfurters and less luncheon meat, sugar and candy, oils and fats. They're eating more chicken, cheese, dark green vegetables and citrus fruits.

Their concern is certainly a step in the right direction, but most still have a way to go, says Paul Lachance, Ph.D., professor of nutrition and food science at Rutgers University, New Brunswick, New Jersey. "The average American doesn't know where the nutrients are. He doesn't go shopping and pick up a vegetable and say, 'Here's my vitamin A, or here's my vitamin C.' He'll read the label on a prepared food, but won't know what it means. When it comes to details, most people just don't know much about nutrition."

And they have misconceptions, contends Phyllis Havens of Hampden, Maine, a registered dietitian and consulting nutritionist. "People think margarine is so much better than butter, but then they'll use twice as much of it, not realizing there's as much fat and calories in it as butter," she says. "And they think granola bars are a healthy snack, when they're actually loaded with fat and sugar."

Ms. Havens is "reeducating" the clients she sees in her private practice and at the Holistic Center in South Portland, using an updated version of an old teaching tool—the four basic food groups. "I am encouraging people to look at them again, as a guide, but with an emphasis on specific nutrients and whole foods—whole grains, low-fat dairy products, fresh fruits, dark green, leafy vegetables and fish and poultry."

Good advice. But why exactly is it that individuals fail to do a good job at personal nutrition? It's not just lack of knowledge, often, but certain patterns of eating, or even patterns of living, that predispose many of us to dietary problems. And these dietary problems can often turn into health problems. Let's look at several common eating patterns or diets and see what's wrong with each. Where are the hidden danger zones and how can they be eliminated?

The High-Protein Predicament

Jean and Jerry like the quick weight-loss diet. It lets them fill up on their favorite foods—steak and shrimp—and still drop five pounds in a week. It also allows them to eat plenty of chicken, low-fat cheese, lean fish and hard-boiled eggs, and to drink as much diet soda and coffee as their kidneys can handle. It prohibits any other foods. No fruits or vegetables. No carbohydrates. It's a diet they go on again and again, every time they regain those five pounds.

What's wrong with this diet? For starters, it's high in fat. Fifty percent or more of its calories come from fat. "Anyone who's worried about heart disease or liver or kidney problems would want to avoid eating this way," Dr. Lachance says. "And it's also higher in sodium than is wise."

Fiber in this diet would be minuscule. "You are begging for dependency on a laxative," Dr. Lachance says. Low fiber intake could aggravate gallstones or diverticulosis, Ms. Havens adds.

Such a diet might not deliver all the calcium you need, and its high protein content would make your body excrete up to twice the calcium it would normally. "Unless you are eating a lot of low-fat dairy products, you could definitely increase the risk of osteoporosis [thin, weak bones], especially with older women, with this diet," Ms. Havens says.

And all the other nutrients that are found mostly in fruits, vegetables and whole grains would be missing in this diet—vitamins C and A, magnesium, potassium and, among the B complex, thiamine, B_6 and folate. "When you see the number of nutrients that aren't being delivered and the health risks involved, you have to ask yourself, 'Why should I use this diet?'" Dr. Lachance says.

Adding insult to injury, much of that exhilaratingly quick

weight loss on the high-protein diet is water, water that gushes back into your body the minute you resume eating carbohydrates. Both nutritionists recommend a reducing diet high in fiber and low in fats. "I recommend a diet similar to the Pritikin diet [high in grains and vegetables, very low in fat], but one that allows about 20 percent fat," Ms. Havens says. Dr. Lachance likes the diet outlined in *The F-* [for fiber] *Plan Diet* (Crown Publishers, 1983).

Both allow you ample quantities of food, while minimizing the most concentrated source of calories—fat.

The Iron Impasse

Let's look at another dieter, Joan, who's proud of her superslim figure and admits she practically lives on a few low-cal staples—cottage cheese, yogurt, broiled chicken and fish, lettuce and tomato, zucchini and string beans. She's also a big tea and coffee drinker. She thinks it helps dull her appetite. And it perks her up. Trouble is, she hasn't been feeling very perky lately.

Joan's big problem is iron. She's getting less than half of what she needs from her food, and her tea and coffee drinking further inhibits absorption of the little she does get, according to Ms. Havens.

"I would put the focus on lots of dark green, leafy vegetables like broccoli, spinach and even some of the more unusual greens like collards, mustard and kale," she says. "And I would try to convince her that some iron-rich legumes like beans and lentils aren't all that fattening. A half cup of cooked kidney beans has only 110 calories."

Dr. Lachance is very concerned about the difficulty of absorbing iron from grains and vegetables. "I'd suggest instead some of the very lean red meats, the muscle meats from the shoulder and rump." Women unwilling to eat much red meat will have to take an iron supplement, he believes.

How about someone who's eating no meat at all?

When they went vegetarian ten years ago, Tom and Tina had the best of intentions and enough information to get them started. They'd read Frances Moore Lappé's *Diet for a Small*

Planet and shifted their preferences toward dairy products, eggs, grains and plenty of fresh fruit and vegetables. They even got to like tofu and miso. They were determined to avoid all the ills associated with an overabundant society—obesity, high blood pressure, heart disease. But were they setting themselves up for unseen troubles?

Both zinc and iron deficiencies can be a problem in a vegetarian diet, especially for women, researchers have found. And vegans, who eat no dairy products or eggs, often get less than the Recommended Dietary Allowance (RDA) for calcium. "No vegetable is a reliable source of zinc, and I'm very supportive of every vegetarian taking a zinc supplement," Ms. Havens says.

"And I think it's worthwhile if they're not feeling the highest energy level possible to have a blood test to see if they are iron deficient," she adds. If they are, she will try adding iron-rich legumes, blackstrap molasses and dark green, leafy vegetables to their diet for three months, then have a second blood test done. If the dietary changes aren't working, she'll then suggest an iron supplement.

Calcium may be less of a problem. A surprising source of calcium can be tofu, when set into curd with calcium carbonate, says Georgene Barte, associate professor of foods and nutrition at Oregon State University, Corvallis. One serving of tofu has about a third the amount of calcium a serving of milk has.

B_{12} used to be considered an inevitable deficiency for strict vegetarians. Now, though, researchers have found significant amounts of B_{12} in cultured and fermented foods like miso, soy sauce and tempeh.

Vegetarians should realize that hard cheeses and nuts can be much higher in fats than lean red meat. One ounce of Cheddar cheese has 9.1 grams of fat; one ounce of lean, trimmed T-bone steak has only 3 grams. An ounce of almonds (about 22 nuts) has 16.4 grams of fat.

"I think vegetarians are more likely to go overboard with fats when they first make the switch, when instead of eating meat, they are eating whole-milk dairy products and eggs," says Ms. Havens. "I'd avoid those 'gourmet' vegetarian cookbooks that emphasize sour cream, cheese and eggs."

How about someone whose problem is a vegetable aversion?

Meat-Eater's Malaise

As far as Frank is concerned, the only vegetable "real men" eat is potatoes—french-fried with a burger, boiled with a pot roast, or hash-browned with eggs. Like the picky little kid he was, Frank finds most fruits and vegetables yucky. But his childish holdover could be making him deficient in vitamins A and E, folate and potassium.

Let's not knock potatoes. A medium baked spud has 844 milligrams of potassium (about a third of the usual daily adult intake), 30 milligrams of vitamin C (half the RDA) and four grams of fiber, about a third of what many people get in a day. The problem is in the way most of us cook potatoes, says Ms. Barte. We peel the nutrient- and fiber-rich skin off, and boil or fry away some of the vitamin C. Frank should be eating a baked potato, skin and all.

And adding even a few choice fruits and vegetables to his limited menu could make the difference between health and deficiency.

"I find that some adults who are really turned off by cooked vegetables do better with raw ones," says Ms. Havens. "If they don't like cooked spinach, I suggest they start eating it raw mixed in with iceberg lettuce, gradually increasing the amount. Or they might enjoy dips with carrots or green pepper strips."

Like many children, some adults dislike strong-flavored vegetables like cabbage, broccoli and onions. Instead, they may enjoy sweet-flavored carrots, winter squash and sweet potatoes, served with a little butter and maple syrup. These vegetables would certainly solve Frank's vitamin A problem. A four-ounce serving of sweet potatoes or carrots would supply his RDA of 5,000 international units (I.U.), as would half a cup of butternut squash.

Citrus fruits and juices would be his best bet for vitamin C. Just one cup of orange juice would give him 124 milligrams of C, and an additional bonus of 496 milligrams of potassium and 500 I.U. of A.

Calcium Countdown

Mary's daughter has been nagging her to get more calcium in her diet ever since Mary broke her wrist in a fall a few years ago. Now she's 70 and unsteady on her feet. Her daughter fears she'll fall down and break a hip one of these days.

The problem is that Mary thinks she gets all the calcium she needs. She gets about a cup of milk a day, with cereal and coffee, and another serving as a slice of cheese or half a cup of cottage cheese. Other foods boost her daily intake to the RDA of 800 milligrams.

But that amount is not enough to prevent osteoporosis, researchers say.

"From what I've read, I think the RDA for women past 30 should be 1,000 milligrams, and for those past menopause, 1,200 to 1,500 milligrams," says Ms. Barte.

Getting that much calcium in your diet would mean getting the equivalent of four or five cups of milk. Each cup has 290 milligrams of calcium, or 34 milligrams per ounce. One big miscalculation is that people think one serving of cottage cheese, normally about a quarter cup, equals the calcium in a cup of milk. It actually takes about two cups of cottage cheese to equal one cup of milk, Ms. Barte says.

The only foods that top dairy products for calcium content are sardines and salmon, but only if you eat the soft small bones mixed in with the flesh. Sardines have 124 milligrams of calcium per ounce; salmon, 73 milligrams.

No Time for Nutrition

What if you're concerned with getting an entire busy family to eat better?

Joan and her family are lucky enough to see one another long enough to nuzzle up and say, "Hello, stranger." Both she and her husband work, and he's on the road a day or two each week. When her two teenage sons aren't in school, they're at band practice or a swimming meet. Joan gave up on sit-down meals when she realized the only family member willing to show up on a regular basis was the dog.

Now meals are whenever you're hungry and whatever you manage to scrounge out of the refrigerator. She tries to keep it stocked with foods the kids like and can easily fix themselves — ground beef, tuna, cheese, eggs, hot dogs and beans, bread, milk, cold cuts, frozen pizza. And, of course, sodas, potato chips and ice cream. Her kids would mutiny if she didn't keep those things around the house. She's about the only one who eats the salad fixings she brings home. She'd like her family to eat better, but where to start?

The dangers in this diet are too much fat and sugar and too little fiber, B and C vitamins, and minerals like magnesium and potassium, Ms. Havens says.

"If she were willing to commit even a few hours a week to cooking, she could make a huge pot of nutritious soup with beans, brown rice and all kinds of vegetables, keep part in the refrigerator and freeze some for use later. I do that myself, and I'm a busy professional."

Planning ahead by making and freezing large batches of other good foods—chili, cornbread, beans (which could later be refried for tacos), pizzas cut up into individual slices—could

AND THE ANSWERS ARE. . .

The four basic food groups are: meat and eggs, dairy products, grains and cereals, and fruits and vegetables.

Romaine has six times as much vitamin A and three times as much calcium and vitamin C as iceberg lettuce.

Brown rice has three times as much fiber and twice as much potassium and riboflavin as white rice.

Nuts, beans, whole grains and green, leafy vegetables are rich in magnesium.

Bananas, oranges, potatoes and tomatoes have lots of potassium.

Meat, whole grains and nuts are good sources of zinc.

The American Health Foundation, a leading nonprofit research group, recommends you get 20 to 25 percent of your calories from fat, 15 percent from protein and 60 to 65 percent from carbohydrates.

Scientists now list between 50 and 60 known nutrients needed by the body.

actually save her time in the long run. And having cut-up crunchies or low-sugar sweets like homemade oatmeal cookies within a hungry hand's reach might help wean her sugar-loving adolescents off their regular fix.

A more realistic solution, says Dr. Lachance, would be to simply supplement the family's fast foods with items to make a complete meal. "If you're eating a hamburger or a pizza, which is not such bad food, make sure you have a salad and a glass of skim milk, too, not a soda," he says.

And you can choose convenience foods with an eye toward more nourishment and less fat and salt. Look for stir-fry meat and vegetable combinations and dieter's dinners, and pick store-brand frozen vegetables without butter or sauces.

Nutritional danger zones can make an unexpected appearance in just about anyone's dietary lifestyle. Sometimes they pop up with a change of schedule; other times they just creep up on us. But once we're aware of them, that's half the battle. And the rest, our nutritionists agree, is not that difficult.

Build Your D-Fence against Aging Bones

He was certain he was about to die. At 82, the infirmities of old age had been limited to a mild case of diabetes and a hip fracture, from which he had recently recovered. Now he found himself back in the hospital, his bones weak and aching from what he was sure was an insidious cancer eating him alive.

Fortunately, his doctor's diagnosis wasn't made in such terrified haste. In fact, this physician even refused to jump to an easy conclusion when the x-rays showed the classic symptoms of osteoporosis: a wasting of bone mass and many collapsed vertebrae. His decision to prescribe vitamin D and calcium was based in part on something his frightened elderly patient told him in conversation—that he avoided sunlight and didn't drink milk or take vitamins.

Uriel A. Barzel, M.D., of New York's Montefiore Medical Center and Albert Einstein School of Medicine, suspected that what he was seeing, x-rays and patient's fears aside, was osteomalacia, an adult version of a now-rare childhood vitamin D deficiency disease called rickets. Both conditions are characterized by painful, thinning bones that, left untreated, can lead to deformities.

Until recently, vitamin D deficiency was thought to be almost as rare as the bubonic plague, eradicated by D-fortified foods such as milk. But in the past few years, researchers and clinicians alike have become concerned that it may be a serious hidden problem among the nation's elderly. One researcher calls it "an unrecognized epidemic," and it may be implicated as a factor in that scourge of old age, hip fracture. What's more, it's often difficult to diagnose, frequently masquerading as that other bone-thinning condition, osteoporosis.

Dr. Barzel took an educated guess with his patient and was proved correct in the best possible way—the man got well in three weeks of treatment with supplements. But, Dr. Barzel acknowledges, it's a diagnosis that's easy to miss.

A Disease in Disguise

"Because vitamin D deficiency is uncommon in the general population, the family physician or internist may fail to consider vitamin D and may miss this diagnosis in the elderly," the physician says. "The symptoms and signs of early vitamin D deficiency may be difficult to recognize. The patient may have weakness, which may be attributed to coexisting disease. Although bone pain is quite specific, it may be mistaken for metastatic disease [cancer] or osteoporosis, not only by the patient but also by the physician."

Though a bone biopsy may tell the most accurate story, Dr. Barzel has advised other physicians to first ask the right questions to pinpoiont whether a patient is getting an adequate amount of D. If not, a short therapeutic trial with moderate amounts of vitamin D and calcium can be diagnosis and cure in one. "The response of the patient is both quick and dramatic and confirms the diagnosis," Dr. Barzel says.

Better diagnostic techniques are imperative, because recent studies give every indication that vitamin D deficiency is not rare. In fact, there may be cause for alarm. Studies of health-conscious and apparently healthy elderly participants showed that at least half got less than the minimum daily requirement of vitamin D—200 international units (I.U.). A third were getting less than 100 I.U. In a study of 142 elderly hip-fracture patients at Massachusetts General Hospital in Boston, 40 percent were D deficient and three-quarters of them had osteomalacia. "As many as 30 to 40 percent of all hip-fracture patients in the United States have osteomalacia," says researcher Samuel H. Doppelt, M.D., of Harvard.

To understand these figures, it's first necessary to understand how vitamin D works. In the body, the raw vitamin is changed into its active form, a hormone known as calcitriol, by the kidneys and the liver. This active form enhances the absorption of calcium to nourish the nerves, muscles and skeleton. Without D, the body begins to literally strip-mine the bones for calcium to meet the needs of the nerves and muscles, leaving the bones thin, brittle and breakable.

In its advanced stages, osteomalacia can be extremely painful and may be accompanied by tetany, muscle spasms that are caused by a calcium imbalance. But even before pain starts, a D deficiency can do enough damage to cripple. It is a hidden epidemic in many ways. "A D deficiency of less severity can cause an accumulated bone loss with age and can be painless until a bone break occurs," says A. Michael Parfitt, M.D., director of the Bone and Mineral Research Laboratory at Henry Ford Hospital in Detroit. "And I'm afraid this is rather common among elderly people."

The reason? Although it is difficult for most of us to avoid getting enough vitamin D, it's even more difficult for elderly people to get enough. It's only abundant in foods that are hardly a staple of the American menu: fatty fish such as mackerel and swordfish. In the United States, it's added to milk, which many elderly people use simply to color tea or coffee. But it's most abundantly supplied when the sun's ultraviolet rays strike the skin, activating a vitamin D precursor. About 90 percent of the major circulating form of D comes from our skin supply. In fact, basking in the sun for about 30 minutes a day is enough to eliminate the need for any dietary D at all in healthy adults.

But, like Dr. Barzel's patient, many elderly people don't get enough sun. They may be housebound by illness or disability, or simply less physically active and less likely to spend time outdoors. But, for whatever reason, they simply don't tap into the most available supply of D there is.

A Place in the Sun

Theoretically, doctors could solve the problem by prescribing cruises to warm, sunny islands or, at the very least, daily strolls in the afternoon sun. A group of British doctors stopped just short of recommending that when they assessed the vitamin D status of 110 men and women nearing retirement age. They extolled the virtues of "a sunny holiday" when they saw what it did to the vitamin D levels of their subjects. Almost all of those who had the highest concentrations of circulating D had been on vacation in sunnier climes, some as long as four months previously. One woman, whose diet was relatively poor in D, nevertheless had the highest concentration of D in her bloodstream. The reason? She had just gotten a two-week dose of sunshine on Malta (*Human Nutrition: Clinical Nutrition,* March, 1984).

But for many, a vacation in the sun simply isn't possible. And the sun isn't always an entirely reliable source of the sunshine vitamin, either. During the winter months, the sun slants its rays through the ozone layer of the atmosphere, which filters out much of the ultraviolet light the skin needs to manufacture D. Studies show that blood levels of the vitamin tend to drop in the winter, especially among elderly women. Urban dwellers may see the sun even less than the housebound, especially if they live and work in the shadows of tall buildings. Pollution may also be a factor. A progressive increase in atmospheric ozone and pollutants between 1951 and 1972 produced a 20 percent decrease in the amount of ultraviolet radiation reaching the earth. Some researchers believe the decrease in ultraviolet light parallels a progressive increase in hip-fracture mortality.

There is another confounding factor. Elderly people also may have faulty vitamin D metabolism—an inability to convert vitamin D into its active form in adequate amounts. Hector DeLuca, Ph.D., chairman of the biochemistry department at the University of Wisconsin in Madison, with his colleagues, was the first to demonstrate that D has to be changed into an active hormonal form before it can function. Since isolating the hormone, Dr. DeLuca and others have been experimenting with ways to use it pharmacologically to treat postmenopausal and old-age osteoporosis.

"In both old age and the postmenopausal state, the vitamin D hormone doesn't respond as it should," says Dr. DeLuca. "Calcium absorption is low, bone turnover—the tearing down of old bone and rebuilding of new bone—is low. If you have low calcium absorption, the body continues to draw on bone calcium to meet nerve and muscle needs. This contributes to the thinning of bones. When they become thin enough, they fracture."

Several recent clinical tests have been "promising," says Dr. DeLuca. Postmenopausal women given small doses of the vitamin D hormone had increased calcium retention in the bones, increased bone mass and a decrease in bone-fracture rates. The hormone works, apparently, because it circumvents the metabolism problem. Giving D alone is ineffective, says Dr. DeLuca.

But if your metabolism is working up to par, and you're in the high-risk category, a supplement may be needed. "Without D, you can't make the hormonal form," says the researcher. "I personally think the best way to get D is by sunlight. But, unlike some other nutrition people, I recommend a multivitamin so you can get all the basic nutrients you need, including D."

If you are taking a D supplement, make sure it's no more than 400 I.U. a day. Vitamin D in larger amounts can be toxic.

"Taking 400 I.U. once a day will keep you well below the level that can cause any harm," says Dr. Parfitt. "When you weigh the possible toxic effects against the dangers of D deficiency, based on present evidence, I'm not convinced of the danger of D toxicity."

Vitamin C
Deficiency Alert

How can you *not* get adequate amounts of vitamin C? Its Recommended Dietary Allowance (RDA) is a mere 60 milligrams a day, and it's found in everything from orange juice to brussels sprouts.

Yet, like a lot of people, you may have a deficit of C without even being aware of it. Your body, though, will know the score. Frequent infections, wounds that take forever to heal, bleeding gums, skin problems—these and other calamities may be your body's way of saying there isn't enough C to go around.

The scarcity occurs when your personal vitamin C economy goes into recession—when your C supply is too low or the C demand is too high. Your supply depends solely on your intake. (Your body can't cook up its own vitamin C—it has to send out.) And your intake may or may not be what it should be. Nutritional surveys show that many people's C intakes don't even meet the RDA. Or, to look at the flip side of the problem, the demands (the forces that can increase your need for vitamin C) may be more numerous than you think. Smoking cigarettes, taking birth control pills, living or working in polluted air, being allergic—such factors may tax your C supply to the limit.

So how do you know if you're sliding into biochemical recession? You take inventory of your C intake and requirements, and assess how they balance out.

And that's where this quiz comes in. First, read through the 19 quiz statements and check off the ones that apply to you. Each represents a vitamin C demand—a factor that may destroy C in your system or accelerate your body's use of C or possibly indicate a need for C to help prevent a medical condition.

Second, follow the instructions in the scoring section to assess your vitamin C intake and to discover how your selected demands compare. This part can't tell you whether you're in a state of vitamin depletion (your doctor must determine that) or how much daily C you should be getting. But it can tell you whether you have a possible vitamin C deficit—whether your C demands could be outpacing your supply.

Check the Statements That Apply to You

1. I'm under a tremendous amount of stress or feel tense or anxious much of the time. (Research shows that people's need for vitamin C greatly increases in stressful situations, and some investigators report that vitamin C has reduced tension and anxiety in several patients.)

2. I take daily doses of aspirin. (Aspirin can block vitamin C from entering the bloodstream.)

3. I don't adjust well to hot or cold environments. (Vitamin C has been used to treat people with heat stress, to help workers adapt to heat and humidity and to enable people to withstand cold weather.)

4. I'm recovering from surgery or have a burn or wound. (Researchers have found that vitamin C is crucial for normal wound repair and may dramatically accelerate healing of bedsores, burns and surgical incisions.)

5. I eat a high-fat, high-cholesterol diet or have elevated cholesterol and triglyceride levels. (Studies from around the world indicate that vitamin C may reduce cholesterol and triglycerides in humans and thus help decrease their risk of heart disease.)

6. I live or work around toxic chemicals or in polluted air. (In human and animal studies, vitamin C has been shown to protect the body against environmental poisons—including the industrial toxins cadmium and benzene, the heavy metal lead and the airborne pollutant ozone.)

☐ **7.** I take birth control pills. (Oral contraceptives seem to reduce concentrations of vitamin C in the body.)

☐ **8.** I have an allergy. (Vitamin C has been shown to alleviate certain allergic reactions, including those brought on by ragweed pollen.)

☐ **9.** I take steroids. (Studies suggest that vitamin C may help reduce the high rate of infection among those who take these drugs.)

☐ **10.** I have weak immunity and suffer from frequent respiratory infections. (Researchers have demonstrated that vitamin C can strengthen the body's resistance to bacterial and viral invaders.)

☐ **11.** I smoke. (Inhaling cigarette smoke may burn up large quantities of vitamin C in the body.)

☐ **12.** I have cancer or have a family history of cancer. (People with higher intakes of vitamin C seem to have lower risks of certain cancers. And with laboratory animals and in the test tube, researchers have established that C is a potent antitumor agent.)

☐ **13.** I'm prone to skin problems. (Increased vitamin C intake has been associated with a lower incidence of minor skin disorders.)

☐ **14.** I suffer frequent urinary infections. (Vitamin C can destroy certain bacteria, including *Escherichia coli,* the most common instigator of urinary tract infections. Thus, doctors have used C to prevent the ailments in people prone to them.)

☐ **15.** I have asthma. (Vitamin C has been shown to relieve some asthmatic symptoms, including attacks.)

☐ **16.** I eat a lot of processed meats, smoked fish or other foods containing nitrates. (Nitrates are often added to foods as preservatives or flavoring and coloring agents. But in the stomach they can be transformed into nitrosamines, potent cancer-causing substances. Research indicates, however, that vitamin C may be able to block this transformation or at least minimize its destructive effects.)

☐ **17.** My gums aren't as healthy as they should be. (Several studies suggest that the condition of the gums can actually be improved with increased intakes of C.)

☐ **18.** I have glaucoma. (The common element in all types of glaucoma is greater-than-normal pressure inside the eyeball. Researchers have demonstrated that oral vitamin C can often decrease this pressure, sometimes dramatically.)

☐ **19.** I'm a diabetic. (Research suggests that vitamin C may be able to improve the body's handling of blood sugar. There's even some evidence that C can inhibit or prevent damage to the walls of blood vessels caused by chronic high blood sugar levels. Diabetics should know, however, that vitamin C may interfere with urinary blood sugar tests.)

WHAT'S YOUR SCORE?

Now you have an idea of how many factors may be drawing on your stores of C.

To evaluate the supply side of the equation, estimate your daily C intake (including supplements) for three consecutive days and take an average. The table on page 70 will help you determine the C content of C-rich foods, and nutritional food labels can give you even more data. Just keep in mind that the cooking and storing of foods can decrease their C content below established values.

The chart below can tell you whether you have a possible vitamin C deficit.

If Your Intake Is	And You Checked	Then You Have
low (up to 100 mg. daily)	at least 1 statement	a possible need for more C
medium (100 to 300 mg. daily)	1 or 2 statements	probably no need for more C
	3 or more statements	a possible need for more C
maximum* (300 or more mg. daily)	5 or fewer statements	probably no need for more C
	6 or more statements	a possible need for more C

*Certain medical conditions may respond to even higher intakes, but such high-dose therapy should be supervised by a qualified medical professional.

FOOD SOURCES OF VITAMIN C

Food	Portion	Vitamin C (mg.)
Orange juice, fresh-squeezed	1 cup	124
Grapefruit juice	1 cup	94
Papaya	½ medium	94
Orange	1	70
Brussels sprouts, raw	4 sprouts	65
Green peppers, raw, chopped	½ cup	64
Cantaloupe	¼	56
Tomato juice	1 cup	45
Strawberries	½ cup	42
Broccoli, raw, chopped	½ cup	41
Grapefruit	½	41
Cauliflower, raw, chopped	½ cup	36
Potato, baked	1 medium	26
Tomato, raw	1	22
Turnip greens, cooked	½ cup	20
Cabbage, raw, chopped	½ cup	17
Blackberries	½ cup	15
Blueberries	½ cup	9
Spinach, raw, chopped	½ cup	8
Cherries, sweet	½ cup	5
Mung bean sprouts	¼ cup	3

SOURCES: Adapted from
Composition of Foods: Vegetables and Vegetable Products, Agriculture Handbook No. 8-11, by Nutrition Monitoring Division (Washington, D.C.: Human Nutrition Information Service, U.S. Department of Agriculture, 1984).
Composition of Foods: Fruits and Fruit Juices, Agriculture Handbook No. 8-9, by Consumer Nutrition Center (Washington, D.C.: Human Nutrition Information Service, U.S. Department of Agriculture, 1982).

Protecting and Restoring Your Good Health

How to Avoid a Dangerous Blood Clot

If you've reached your fifties or sixties, chances are you've probably got some fatty buildup inside your arteries. In fact, if you've been living the typical American lifestyle and eating the typical American diet all these years, chances are pretty good that you've got a significant degree of atherosclerosis. Sure, you'll want to do all you can to keep the plaque lining your arteries from getting worse. But if preventing a heart attack is your goal, you'll also want to do everything you can to prevent a blood clot.

"There was a lot of controversy over the years as to whether or not blood clots were the primary mechanism for people developing heart attacks," Salvatore V. Pizzo, M.D., Ph.D., associate professor of pathology and biochemistry at Duke University Medical Center, told us. "And the answer now seems to be unequivocally yes. Certainly 80 percent of heart attacks are the result of having blood clots develop on top of blood vessels that are diseased. But if you don't have a clot, you generally don't get a heart attack. So anything that promotes dissolving clots clearly would be protective against heart attacks," he says.

In a study by Dr. Pizzo and his co-workers, it was found that moderate exercise enhanced fibrinolytic (clot-dissolving) activity (*New England Journal of Medicine,* May 1, 1980). "We measured a protein called plasminogen activator," says

Dr. Pizzo. "It's a protein in the blood vessel walls that gets released whenever blood starts to clot. It's one of the major ways we dissolve a blood clot.

"Plasminogen is a protein that's in the blood all the time in an inactive form. When plasminogen activator gets released from vessel walls, it converts plasminogen to plasmin, which actually dissolves a clot. No activator—no plasmin—no dissolution of the clot.

"So the point is, if you have a damaged vessel which is prone to clot, and it starts to clot, what may determine whether or not that process continues until it obstructs the vessel is whether or not the plasminogen activator levels are high enough."

One thing that raises the level of plasminogen activator is exercise. "In people with very low levels of this protein—people at fairly high risk for developing blood clots—we found that levels went up about 250 percent following a ten-week physical conditioning program," Dr. Pizzo told us. "That put them in the range with people who have a much lower risk of developing blood clots." The exercise program, which is considered moderate, consisted of 45 minutes of jogging, three times a week.

"Certainly moderate exercise is to be recommended in people who are in reasonable health," says Dr. Pizzo. "If there is any question at all, however, people should consult their doctor before they start exercising."

Something Fishy

Another way to help fend off a fatal blood clot is by making a few additions to your diet. For instance, doctors have linked the low incidence of heart attacks among Greenland Eskimos to their consumption of lots of fish.

The active ingredient, they've found, is a fatty acid called EPA, short for eicosapentanoic acid. One way it exerts its influence is through its effect on platelets, those disk-shaped elements in the blood that clump together at the site of a wound to stanch the flow of blood. The problems begin when platelets become excessively "sticky" and clump together, or aggregate, at the wrong times, blocking the vital flow of blood through an artery.

When West German researchers fed subjects a diet whose

sole source of protein and fat was mackerel, a fish rich in EPA, for one week, their platelets aggregated much less. And the formation of thromboxane, a powerful clumping agent made by the body, was also reduced (*Lancet,* March 1, 1980).

In another West German study, volunteers ate their normal diet supplemented with three tablespoons of cod-liver oil daily for 25 days. Cod-liver oil is also rich in EPA. The subjects' bleeding time increased, which is an indication of a lesser propensity to clot. Their number of platelets, platelet aggregation and thromboxane formation all decreased significantly (*Circulation,* March, 1983).

Just how does EPA work? Dale E. Hammerschmidt, M.D., associate professor of medicine at the University of Minnesota Medical School in Minneapolis, explains that when platelets are stimulated, they release a substance called arachidonic acid, which leads to the production of thromboxane. A diet high in EPA, however, results in platelets that release EPA when stimulated, which leads to the production of an analog of thromboxane that is only about one-tenth as potent, so there's much less chance of a clot forming.

Now, a mackerel diet may sound fine to Eskimos, but you may find it a little hard to swallow. And three tablespoons of cod-liver oil is an excessive dose, containing exceptionally large amounts of vitamins A and D. You can still do your heart good, though, by increasing your intake of fish rich in EPA— salmon, trout, mackerel, haddock and sardines.

Anticlotting Cuisine

You know what onions and garlic can do for your cooking, but did you know that these pungent edibles can also help prevent blood clots? Arun K. Bordia, M.D., of the department of medicine and cardiology at the Ravindra Nath Tagore Medical College in Udaipur, India, found that garlic increases the fibrinolytic activity of the blood. When Dr. Bordia and his co-workers gave garlic to patients within 24 hours of their suffering a heart attack, they found the fibrinolytic activity increased by 63 percent after 10 days and by 95 percent after 20 days. When they gave garlic to people with no history of heart problems, their fibrinolytic activity rose to 130 percent (*Atherosclerosis,* October, 1977).

That garlic and onions can inhibit platelet aggregation has been shown in several studies. Acting on that information, Amar N. Makheja, Ph.D., and his associates, of the department of biochemistry at George Washington University School of Medicine in Washington, D.C., set out to identify the active compounds.

"I had been looking at the effects of aspirin and similar drugs on platelets and thromboxane," Dr. Makheja told us. "Being Indian, I knew of the folklore about onions and garlic. And a lot of the research work was done in India. But there was no explanation of *why* onion and garlic block platelet aggregation, and I thought maybe I could find a reason."

He found that onions and garlic, "commonly used in the diet, contain chemically similar compounds which inhibit platelet aggregation by blocking thromboxane synthesis" (*Lancet*, April 7, 1979).

"Onions and garlic don't have a permanent effect on the blood platelets," explains Dr. Makheja. "After several hours the effect will disappear, so you'd have to eat them every day. But you will get some benefit and there's no harm."

Just how potent are onions and garlic? A researcher at Radcliffe Infirmary in Oxford, England, found that eating just four cloves of garlic *completely* inhibited platelet aggregation induced by a clumping agent 1 hour after ingestion. Like Dr. Makheja, though, he found that the inhibitory effects disappeared about 2½ hours after ingestion (*Lancet,* April 4, 1981). But onions and garlic weren't created equal. According to Dr. Makheja, 3½ ounces of garlic has about five times the activity of an equal amount of onions.

More Fancy Food Work

Dr. Hammerschmidt is responsible for discovering the anti-aggregatory effects of Chinese black tree fungus, commonly used in Chinese cooking. While studying a related topic, Dr. Hammerschmidt used his own platelets and found that they refused to aggregate, even when exposed to what he called "industrial-strength stimuli." He eventually determined that the Chinese mushrooms, eaten the night before, were the cause (*Journal of the American Medical Association,* January 15, 1982). Dr. Makheja later confirmed that observation when he identified the specific antiplatelet substance contained in the mushrooms.

In Thailand, doctors have reported that capsicum, or hot pepper, a usual ingredient in Thai meals, increases fibrinolytic activity. Say the doctors, "Although the enhanced fibrinolytic effect of capsicum appears for only a short duration, . . . one may expect that in those people who ingest capsicum with their meals, the fibrinolytic activity would be [stimulated] . . . several times a day. This daily stimulation. . . is perhaps sufficient to prevent thromboembolism [blood clot] among the majority of such consumers. Capsicum ingestion may be a factor contributing to the low incidence of thromboembolism in Thais." The doctors also point out that capsicum in normal amounts causes no harm to the stomach lining (*American Journal of Clinical Nutrition,* June, 1982).

Clot Prevention Made E-C

Vitamins E and C may also help prevent blood clots. Manfred Steiner, M.D., Ph.D., director of the division of hematology/oncology at the Memorial Hospital in Pawtucket, Rhode Island, and professor of medicine at Brown University, has studied the effects of vitamin E and aspirin on platelets.

In a study of normal, healthy individuals, Dr. Steiner measured the effect on platelets of taking vitamin E, aspirin, or vitamin E *and* aspirin. "Aspirin has been shown to inhibit platelet aggregation," Dr. Steiner told us. "Vitamin E also inhibits platelet aggregation to a lesser degree. But there's one thing vitamin E does that aspirin does not do—it reduces the adherence of platelets to collagen.

"In our scheme of thinking about the development of an arterial thrombus, we think of platelets adhering to a vessel wall that has been damaged—where the continuity of the endothelial cells (the cells lining the inside of the arteries) has been broken and subendothelial tissue is exposed. So first comes adherence of the platelets to the vessel wall, then the process of platelet aggregation sets in. Vitamin E inhibits the platelets' adherence to collagen in a test tube—a situation similar to a damaged blood vessel in the body. We think it will have the same effect in the vessel wall," says Dr. Steiner.

"Animal studies have clearly shown that vitamin E protects the endothelial cells. It allows them to continue to produce a substance called prostacyclin in good amounts. Prostacyclin has the opposite effect of thromboxane—it discourages platelet aggregation. When you have an animal that is deficient in vitamin E, prostacyclin production decreases very much. But it is restored by giving the animal vitamin E."

Research indicates that vitamin C is helpful, too. In one study, patients receiving two grams of C daily were shown to have less adhesive platelets. And in tests with patients suffering from heart disease, vitamin C increased the fibrinolytic activity by over 60 percent. Interestingly, none of the patients were deficient in vitamin C.

"The list of individual observations is almost endless," says Dr. Hammerschmidt. "But the message is a simple one: Many of the things we do or eat have important influences on [platelet] function; further study of these phenomena may generate insights that will allow their modification to our benefit."

Clot Causers

There are lots of things you can do to help sidestep a blood clot, but there are also some things you should avoid. "Way out ahead of anything else bad is smoking cigarettes," says Dr. Hammerschmidt. "It puts platelets on a hair trigger. And in people who are susceptible, smoking can cause blood vessels to constrict fairly severely. That can make a blood vessel small enough that it's easier to plug up.

"You almost can't say 'stop smoking' too strongly as a piece of advice, even in people who've already had a heart attack. Their life expectancy is shortened by half if they continue to smoke. And none of this seems to be much influenced by smoking low-tar, low-nicotine cigarettes. The presumably safer cigarettes are quite a long way short of being shown to be any safer than ordinary cigarettes," he says.

Taking birth control pills also increases the risk of a blood clot. "It has been suggested that physicians get written consent from any smoker put on estrogen-containing birth control pills," Dr. Hammerschmidt told us. "If somebody does both, that puts them in a particularly high risk group."

A diet high in saturated fat is also best avoided, because it raises both cholesterol and triglyceride levels. "People who have high cholesterol and triglyceride levels in their blood also have platelets that are more aggregable and stick more to vessel walls," Dr. Hammerschmidt points out. "Diet isn't the major determinant of those levels, but it can make as much as a 20 percent difference."

A Role for Aspirin?

There's been a lot of talk lately about aspirin preventing blood clots. Why aspirin? "The reason people give aspirin to prevent thrombosis is that it acts to block an enzyme in platelets that produces thromboxane, which makes other platelets clump together and causes blood vessels to constrict," says Garret A. FitzGerald, M.D., of the division of clinical pharmacology at Vanderbilt University in Nashville. "That's thought to be very important in the initiation of thrombosis.

"The problem is that the same enzyme it blocks is also present in blood vessel walls. And in blood vessel walls the major product of that enzyme is not thromboxane but prostacyclin, which has precisely the opposite effect: It unclumps platelets and dilates blood vessels. So theoretically, if you give aspirin in a way that hits both the platelet enzyme and the blood vessel wall enzyme, it could limit the benefit to be derived from aspirin in preventing thrombosis—while knocking out thromboxane, which is desirable, you're also knocking out prostacyclin, which would be undesirable."

It sounds like a dead end. But actually, new experiments with low doses of aspirin have been promising. Why is less better? For several reasons.

"Platelets are not complete cells," explains Dr. Hammerschmidt. "So once you've inhibited the enzyme in platelets with aspirin, they're done for. They can't make new enzymes to replace the enzyme that's been inactivated. And it takes a few days to get enough good platelets back to overcome the effect. But the endothelial cells that line the blood vessel walls *can* make new enzymes. So when their enzyme is inactivated, within a matter of hours they'll have made new stuff and be back to normal. So the idea of giving aspirin in very small doses gives you a separation in how well it works on the two cell types."

There's also some data that suggests that the platelet enzyme might be more sensitive to inhibition by aspirin than the enzyme in the blood vessel wall.

Even more encouraging, though, is a study by Dr. FitzGerald and an associate, which showed that there may be a way of administering aspirin so that it prevents thromboxane formation while sparing the vascular capacity to produce prostacyclin (*New England Journal of Medicine,* November 8, 1984). "One way of doing that with aspirin, which is the most potent platelet inhibitory drug that's available to us at the moment, is by taking advantage of the way aspirin is handled in the body," explains Dr. FitzGerald.

"In the liver, aspirin is broken down to a metabolite called salicylate, which has little or no action on the enzyme in platelets and blood vessel walls. But the liver can remove only so much of the drug. So if you give a small enough dose of aspirin, it will be broken down completely and only the inactive metabolite will escape from the liver out into the general circulation. So you prevent the vast bulk of your blood vessel walls from any exposure to aspirin."

Your platelets, however, will still be exposed. "One difference between platelets and blood vessel walls is that platelets circulate," says Dr. FitzGerald. "So as the aspirin passes through the blood vessels leading from the stomach to the liver, it comes in contact with platelets. Because repeated exposure to aspirin has a cumulative effect, by giving aspirin slowly, in very low doses, you can theoretically completely inhibit the platelet enzyme while largely sparing the blood vessel enzyme from exposure to the drug."

In Dr. FitzGerald's study, dosages as low as 20 milligrams (the amount in one-quarter of a children's aspirin tablet) still inhibited thromboxane production. But Dr. FitzGerald stresses that the optimum dosage and timetable for administering aspirin have yet to be determined. Some doctors are already prescribing aspirin to their patients over 40 as a preventive measure. But Dr. FitzGerald remains cautious. "This is pretty frontier stuff right now. There's no evidence as far as the general public that taking aspirin in any way, shape or form prevents heart attacks if they've never had any problems that way before. There's evidence showing that in people who have chest pains, their likelihood of developing a heart attack is diminished. And there's some evidence in people that have suffered a heart attack that aspirin may diminish their risk of having a subsequent one. But there's no evidence yet, because it's a difficult thing to test, that prophylactically taking aspirin has any effect at all."

17 Natural Ways to Boost Your Energy

Richard Curtis may have done what hitherto has been thought impossible. He may have discovered a perpetual-motion machine: himself.

In the morning he teaches creative writing and journalism at a private boys' school in Connecticut. In the afternoon, he's a chimney sweep—The Sultan of Soot, as he's listed in the Yellow Pages. At night, he grades papers, books chimney-cleaning appointments and attends committee meetings. In his spare time, he is a competitive rower and coach, he's a writer (one book published, two more on the way), and he's teaching himself to play the piano.

In short, Richard Curtis usually wrings 20 waking hours out of each day, sleeping catnap-style for only about 4. It's a schedule that would leave most of us with eyelids permanently at half-mast, but Richard Curtis says he never runs out of energy.

"I love it," he says. "I keep discovering something else that fascinates me. I never stop to think if I have the energy for it. When you love something, it creates its own energy. In fact, your energy level can depend on how much you love life in general. I mean, if you're at a good party, you don't leave when it's still going great."

There are some who would say Richard Curtis is a genetic

anomaly, a man who marches to the ticking of a different clock. And they would be right—in part. "We all come with different energy levels," says Charles Kuntzleman, Ed.D., author of *Maximum Personal Energy* (Rodale Press, 1981). "Some people have God-given high-level energy even though they do everything wrong, just as some people are born beautiful and some are born average."

It's true that Richard Curtis is the recipient of some genetic good fortune. But that's not his only edge. He improves on what nature gave him by leading a full, active life, doing things he loves. He has a good reason to get up in the morning and a good reason not to be in such a hurry to go to bed at night.

Like Richard Curtis, you can improve on your genetic programming. You may not be able to go from a shuffle to a sprint, but you can quicken your step. And you can start right now.

Lead the Active Life ● It's the best lesson you can learn from Richard Curtis: Energy begets energy. Don't give in to boredom and malaise. Get up and do something you really want to do, even if you think you're too tired to do it. You'll be amazed at how much energy you really have. "Love is energy, being creative is energy, health is energy," says Harold H. Bloomfield, M.D., author of *The Holistic Way to Health and Happiness* (Simon and Schuster). "The more good things you do for yourself, the more energetic you're going to be." In fact, the very act of *doing* can help you shake the ennui that made you tired in the first place.

Get Physical ● A regular aerobic workout, one that gets your pulse rate galloping, won't poop you out. It'll actually pump you up. You'll have more oxygen-carrying hemoglobin in your red blood cells. Your heart will eject more blood with each beat so it has to work less to circulate it through your body. Your skeletal muscles will gain a greater capacity to use oxygen, and your muscle cells will be better able to burn fats as fuel. With your trained muscles able to use oxygen more efficiently, your breathing rate drops, so you won't get winded so easily. In fact, your whole body will work so efficiently you'll have even more energy to expend. Not only that, studies have shown that regular exercise can help you beat stress, one of life's biggest energy zappers.

Take a Minibreak ● When your motor's about to die on the expressway, you rev it up. When you're about to die at your desk at quarter of three in the afternoon, you've got to put a figurative pedal to the metal. Get up! Remind your body that it's awake. Do a few tension-relieving exercises, advises Dr. Kuntzleman. Shrug your shoulders, roll your head or, better yet, do a lap around the office, the building or the block.

Know Thyself ● Schedule tough jobs for when you're at your energy peak. If you're full of spit and polish in the morning, don't tackle the Great American Novel at ten o'clock at night, after a busy day at the office. If you're a night owl, don't set your alarm for an early start on refinishing the kitchen cabinets. Listen to the ticking of your own biological clock, say the experts. Otherwise you'll wind up fatigued from all that swimming upstream.

Escape from the Sugar Trap ● Sure, sugar gives you a jolt, but you pay for it later. A burst of sugar flooding your bloodstream cues the body to secrete insulin, which rounds the sugar up for storage. Pretty soon, your sugar high becomes a sugar low. If you want more than a manic-depressive reaction from an energy food, choose complex carbohydrates that are released into the bloodstream at a slower rate. You'll be sacrificing a short burst for staying power.

Lose Weight ● Picture yourself climbing two flights of stairs with a bowling ball under each arm. It would be a lot easier without them, wouldn't it? If you're overweight, you're doing roughly the equivalent every time you exert yourself. "Physically carrying 30 to 40 extra pounds is going to make you more fatigued," says Dr. Kuntzleman.

That's just common sense. But obesity loads you with a weight of a different kind. "It can wear you out psychologically, too," he says. "It affects your perception of yourself, making you self-conscious, which is energy draining. You're always mentally defending yourself: 'Hey, I'm okay; my waistline's just a little big.' "

Try a New Twist: Yoga ● "Yoga doesn't magically give you energy," says Swami Saradananda, director of the Sivanda Yoga Vedanta Center in New York. "What it does is release the energy you have by releasing pent-up tension in the body. Tension is basically energy that's blocked. When you release it, you make the energy you have usable."

'Om' Is Where the Heart Is ● When a group of researchers at Harvard and Beth Israel Hospital in Boston tested the effects of relaxation exercises on the sympathetic nervous system of experimental subjects, they discovered something remarkable. Simply sitting quietly in a relaxed position with your eyes closed, repeating a simple word over and over again while shutting off distracting thoughts can reduce the body's response to stress (*Science,* January 8, 1982).

"It's now being shown by science that this state of 'restful alertness' you achieve through meditation is the optimum state of functioning," says Dr. Bloomfield, who is also director of psychiatry at North County Holistic Health Center in Del Mar, California.

Meditation can help you achieve the seemingly impossible: You can be perfectly relaxed and invigorated at the same time.

Take a Shower ● Hot, warm, cold; it doesn't matter. It's the falling water that gives you the kick. There's a little something special in the air around falling water. It's called a negative ion. Scientifically, it's just a molecule that's adopted an extra electron. But for the 30 percent of the population who are ion sensitive, it's nature's little upper. According to laboratory studies, higher concentrations of negative ions in the air lower the levels of a brain chemical called serotonin, which in turn makes us more cheerful and energetic.

Check Your Iron Levels ● Your body uses iron to help manufacture hemoglobin, a protein in red blood cells that carries oxygen to all your tissues and cells. Deprived of that oxygen, your cells—and you—will soon be running on empty. Menstruating women and people over 65 are particularly prone to iron deficiency, which, even before it becomes full-blown anemia, can lead to chronic, foot-dragging fatigue. Iron is abundant in meats, especially beef liver, and to a lesser extent in foods like sunflower seeds, broccoli, apricots, almonds and raisins.

Grab a Handful of Nuts ● If you're feeling fatigued, especially after a strenuous exercise program, you may have what one medical expert calls the mineral blues—a deficiency of potassium and magnesium in muscle cells. Both minerals can be lost through sweat. When stores drop below normal, even a mild deficiency can bring on fatigue. Both potassium and magnesium are abundant in nuts and soybeans. You'll also find potassium plentiful in fruits and vegetables and magnesium in grains and nuts.

Take C and See ● Several medical studies have suggested that people whose diets are lacking in vitamin C grow fatigued more quickly than those whose C intakes are high. There's a bonus with C. It also helps increase your absorption of dietary iron, sometimes as much as 300 percent. But don't pop C—or any other nutrient supplement, for that matter—expecting it to act like a pep pill. It will only have its energizing effect if your lack of energy is the result of a nutrient lack.

Eat a Light Lunch ● It's two o'clock in the afternoon and you and the pile of work on your desk have slid into a mirror-image slump. What happened? You might review your lunch menu. If you ate a heavy meal, you're the victim of postprandial dip, characterized by a drop in body temperature, blood sugar, work efficiency and mood. In many countries, lunch is followed by a siesta. If you can't get a daily nap written into your benefit package, most experts advise eating a light meal—raw veggies or salads—at noon.

Eat a Good Breakfast ● Depending on how much you toss and turn, you can use up 500 to 600 calories getting a good night's sleep. Even if you don't wake up hungry, your body has still been depleted of the vitamins and minerals that give you the energy to tackle a brand-new day. If you don't eat breakfast, warns Max M. Novich, M.D., coauthor of *The High Energy Diet for Dynamic Living* (Grosset and Dunlap), you're likely to "drag along" all morning, feeling tired and headachy and with a touch of low blood sugar.

Make Upbeat Friends ● Did you ever get trapped in a conversation with a chronic griper? As each complaint drones into your consciousness, you feel yourself turning to lead, cell by cell. Unhappy, unpleasant people are downers who sap your energy. You can't avoid them entirely, short of taking up residence in a cave. The next best thing is to make them the minority in your circle of acquaintances. Fill your life with energetic, upbeat people, and you'll be known by the company you keep. "People who love, have fun and care give you good feelings about yourself and your energy levels," says Dr. Kuntzleman.

Give Yourself Something to Look Forward To ● Anticipation of good things to come can give you a burst of energy that can very nearly rouse you out of a coma. That sense of excitement is like "an amphetamine response," says Michael Liebowitz, M.D., author of *The Chemistry of Love* (Little, Brown and Co., 1983). "When we are looking forward to things, especially when pursuing a valued goal, we liven up, have more energy and concentrate better."

Get Away from It All ● You'll learn the secret of this energy booster when you get back from it. Taking a vacation—whether it's skiing in the Alps or boating on the local lake—is a surefire way to recharge.

"The reason is pretty simple," says ball-of-fire Richard Curtis, who explored the vacation phenomenon in his book *Taking Off* (Harmony Books, 1981). "Getting away from it all gets you out of your rut. Putting some distance between yourself and whatever you're working on makes you feel relaxed. In addition to physically separating yourself from your problems, you're opening yourself up to other things. Essentially you're taking your mind off one thing and putting it on something else. When you come back, you've gotten yourself into the mode of seeing new things. You begin to see your life in a new context, and that's invigorating."

Healing That Hernia

When Harold Foley was a boy on his father's farm, it was not unusual for him to hoist and carry a 250-pound burlap bag full of wheat. And as a man, weighing 230 pounds and standing six feet tall, the 44-year-old Foley, a maintenance man at a textile plant in Pennsylvania, could still lift and carry tables and desks by himself.

It was ironic then, when a five-gallon can of paint "gave him," as it is said, a hernia. While stretching over the lower half of a Dutch door to pick up the can, he felt something "pop" in his abdomen and experienced a sharp pain on both sides of his groin.

Within a week the pain was gone, leaving a small bulge below his belt. But Foley ignored the condition until a few weeks later when, during a physical exam for a new job, a doctor discovered the rupture and advised surgery. "I never thought it could have been a hernia," Foley says.

Like this man, most people have only a vague notion of what a hernia is until they experience one themselves.

Put simply, hernia is a general term that describes what happens when a body part goes where it isn't supposed to. In most cases, it means that a corner of the peritoneum, a sac that envelops the intestines and abdominal cavity, has slipped into one of the openings that leads from the abdomen to the chest or legs. (Imagine a tire with a hole in it. Then picture the inner tube poking through the hole and forming a bubble. The "inner tube" is the peritoneum, and the "bubble" is the hernia.)

The most common hernia by far is the inguinal hernia. It is usually found in men. On either side of the groin there is a ring through which, in men, the spermatic cord passes on its way from the abdomen to the scrotum. When a part of the peritoneum protrudes through the ring, down what is called the inguinal canal and into the scrotum, that is an inguinal hernia. Very similar is the femoral hernia, where the peritoneum protrudes into the thigh. It is more common in women than in men.

The second most common form of hernia is the diaphragmatic, or hiatal, hernia. It happens when a section of the intestine or stomach pushes upward, like a germinating plant, through a gap in the diaphragm and into the chest cavity. Other, less common, hernias are found in newborns and pregnant women. A hernia may also occur at the site of a scar from an operation.

Several things can cause a hernia. Most doctors agree that heredity plays a role. Some people are born with hernias or with big inguinal rings, while others have smaller rings. Doctors also blame evolution for hernia. Hernia might be the price we pay for walking upright, they say—in the sense that gravity pulls the abdomen down toward the inguinal rings. "Anatomically, we have an inborn weakness," one physical therapist told us.

Being overweight, though it will not create a hernia, can make matters worse. Obesity stretches the peritoneum like a balloon, making it more likely to pop. "With severe obesity, you get much higher levels of intra-abdominal pressure, which increases the risk of hernia," says Lloyd Nyhus, M.D., a University of Illinois surgeon and author.

"About half of our patients are overweight to the point where we ask them to lose weight," says Donald Welsh, M.D., a surgeon at the Shouldice Hospital in Toronto, a specialty hospital where about 7,000 hernias are repaired every year.

Weak Muscles

Some doctors say that weak abdominal muscles raise the risk of hernia because they don't act as a natural truss, the way strong muscles do. One doctor believes that weak abdominal muscles, and the hernias they cause, are a symptom of our sedentary modern lifestyle.

"In this age of push buttons and mechanical devices that

spare physical effort, one notes a steadily increasing deterioration in the muscular development of man," says Robert E. Rothenberg, M.D., of the Downstate Medical Center in New York. "It is not strange that the less physically active office worker or businessman of today is not as well equipped to withstand these muscular strains as was his hardworking great-grandfather of days gone by."

It is true that even those with strong abdominal muscles— athletes, for example—also suffer hernias, but those who are out of shape still are relatively worse off. "If you took 1,000 men who have sedentary jobs and are overweight and compared them to 1,000 men in good physical condition, you would find more hernias in the first group," says Robert G. Schneider, M.D., staff physician at Norwalk Hospital, an affiliate of Yale University.

Age can also be a factor in hernia. The elderly lose the elasticity and strength of their abdominal muslces, increasing the chance that pressure from within will find a weak spot. Heavy lifting, coughing, straining to move the bowels and childbirth are other kinds of stress that can increase intra-abdominal pressure and trigger a rupture.

Once someone has experienced a hernia, he or she has several options. Surgery is one of them. Hernia repair is one of the ten most common surgical procedures performed by doctors in the United States. Inguinal hernias are the leader, with about 500,000 a year. Hiatal hernias are extremely common, but often go undetected. If they are detected, they can often be managed without surgery.

Not surprisingly, surgery is usually recommended by surgeons. "If you take your hernia to a general surgeon, he will urge you to have it repaired as soon as possible," says Dr. Schneider, author of the book *When to Say No to Surgery* (Prentice-Hall, 1982). "He will tell you that it is best to act now, before it gets bigger, while you are still in good enough health to withstand an operation and before heart disease complicates things." Above all, surgeons will advise that surgery be done before the hernia becomes "incarcerated."

Incarceration happens when the contents of the hernial sac get trapped inside the bubble formed by the peritoneum.

Blood flow to that area can be pinched off, causing what is called strangulation, and the tissue may become infected. The infection may spread and become life-threatening. As with a burst appendix, emergency surgery must be performed. Incarceration is, on the whole, a rarity, but 4,000 people die of strangulated hernias a year in this country, usually because they neglect to seek the right care in time.

Given the risks of not operating, there are also risks to operating. According to Dr. Schneider, 7 of every 100 hernia-surgery patients incur complications such as heart attack, pneumonia, phlebitis, urinary tract infections and blood clots in the lungs.

But a hernia operation may not always provide permanent relief.

"There's a feeling that the operation fixes the problem for all time, when there is actually a 7 percent recurrence rate after three years," says Dr. Schneider. "And I would say that those who have had hernia repairs are more likely to have a rupture than the average person." Others say that the recurrence rate can be as high as 30 percent, and that obesity or age increases the likelihood of a recurrence.

Is Surgery Needed?

At any rate, most hernias come under the heading of elective surgery, which means that there is adequate time after the diagnosis to consider the pros and cons of surgery. There are several things to keep in mind.

"Individuals with a hernia have to assess how big it is and whether it slips back into place when they lie on their backs. They've got to estimate the state of their health, their age and their occupation. They've really got to take the time to think about it, to get a second opinion, to read up on it and maybe get in touch with a network of people who've had hernias," says Dr. Schneider. Surgery is called for, he thinks, only if the hernia is "enormous" and "interferes with a person's life or work to an extraordinary degree." He advises against surgery when there is only a "threat" or a "potential" for hernia.

One alternative to surgery is the truss. Trusses don't cure hernias, but they will press the protruding tissue back into the abdomen. Trusses are best suited to people who aren't called upon to do heavy lifting or strenuous exercise, and for elderly patients who are at high risk for surgery. In recent years, trusses have become more convenient to wear.

"When people think about trusses, they think about the heavy, awkward devices that their fathers or grandfathers wore," says Dr. Schneider. "But the new trusses are like wide elastic bandages that wrap around the abdomen. They're lighter and more comfortable, and they don't need to be worn all the time."

Trusses aren't entirely risk free. They are a temporary measure, not a permanent solution. Their presence doesn't guarantee that the hernia won't strangulate. As people get older, trusses aren't as effective, and trusses shouldn't be worn during the weeks preceding hernia surgery.

A truss should never be worn so tightly that it leaves a mark on the skin, doctors say. Tightness can cause skin damage and may damage the tissue under the skin, thus complicating the matter. Special care has to be taken to prevent the truss from putting pressure on major arteries near the groin.

Hiatal hernias, it's important to point out, are seldom operated on and don't require a truss. The most common symptom of hiatal hernia is heartburn, which can be treated with antacids. Losing weight and slightly elevating the head of the bed sometimes help, too. If a physician advises you to have your hiatal hernia operated on, get a second opinion from a gastroenterologist. Surgery for this kind of hernia should only be a last resort.

Eat More Fiber

Although hernias don't customarily give any warning before they strike, there are measures that people can take to prevent them. Those who are elderly, overweight or have heavy lifting jobs should take special care to keep their weight down and increase their fiber intake.

Weight, of course, creates pressure on the lower abdomen, increasing the chance that the peritoneum will slide into the inguinal ring or find a weak spot in the abdominal wall. Fiber is important because it prevents constipation. Constipation is usually accompanied by straining to move the bowels, and that strain can increase intra-abdominal pressure, which in turn can lead to a hernia.

Cigarette smoking, like eating too little fiber, has an indirect effect on hernia. Cigarettes promote coughing; coughing can trigger a rupture by raising intra-abdominal pressure.

If a person elects to undergo surgery, he or she may discover that the medical procedures involved have changed a lot in the past few years. Not so long ago, hernia patients were confined to a hospital bed for a week or two, and during surgery they were placed under general anesthesia. Today, however, younger patients with uncomplicated hernias often go home the same day they are operated on and are given only local or partial anesthesia. Even those with complications—usually elderly patients, those with heart disease or those who have had an adverse reaction to anesthesia—may stay in the hospital for only three days.

Patients today are also less coddled by their doctors. People are still advised by their physicians to avoid activities such as jogging, shoveling snow or lifting boxes for four to six weeks after the operation. But now they are urged to get out of bed and start taking walks almost immediately after going home. This advice is intended as much to raise a patient's morale and confidence, doctors say, as it is to tone up muscles.

A Metabolic Perk-Up Plan

If you're overweight, you know it's no small injustice. Your reed-slim friend can win a pie-eating contest and not gain an ounce. You, on the other hand, seem to put on five pounds just thinking about pie.

You have a sneaking suspicion that your metabolism is out of whack, but you don't dare suggest it. Most medical experts regard "It's my metabolism" as a lame coverup for all those second helpings you obviously helped yourself to and the chocolate bars they're sure you've stashed in the glove compartment of your car.

But these days they're not so quick to prescribe a diet and

a dose of guilt. It truly may not be your fault. Recent studies, still controversial, indicate that all metabolisms are not created equal. Your skinny pie-eating friend may have a metabolism that allows her to burn up all those excess calories as heat while yours stores them as fat.

Don't be alarmed, though. You're not doomed. There's evidence you can get your metabolism revved up by new patterns and combinations of exercise, diet and everyday habits. Why? To take advantage of a still-mysterious metabolic phenomenon called dietary-induced thermogenesis.

Though quite a mouthful, it simply means that your body generates heat after you've eaten. That's why you often push away from a large meal feeling uncomfortably warm. You can get that same feeling after vigorous exercise, and, of course, that's no coincidence. Something similar is happening.

When you exercise, your body is burning up calories. The digestive process is a calorie-burning activity, too. After a meal the body works hard to store what you've eaten as fuel. Though it retains some food energy as fat, it gives off some as heat. And the more you burn off as heat, the less you store as fat.

Some of the latest research has shown that overweight people many times do not eat more than their thinner counterparts. They simply have sluggish metabolisms that don't generate that slimming after-dinner blaze. And dieting doesn't help. Their efficient, fat-storing metabolisms regard even a moderate caloric cutback as a signal that starvation is at hand and begin to store fat in case the food shortage goes on indefinitely.

Fan Your Fire

But here's the real news. Exercise can fan the flames of even a "sluggish" metabolism—in at least four different ways. The *timing* of your meals and your exercise can also help your slimming program.

Peter M. Miller, Ph.D., director of the Hilton Head Health Institute, South Carolina, teaches his clients to pare the pounds off by fanning those fires. The double whammy of *The Hilton Head Metabolism Diet* (Warner Books, 1983) is a low-calorie but four-meal-a-day diet and moderate but well-timed exercise.

The aim of the Hilton Head Diet is to get those fires stoked and keep them burning all day long. Dr. Miller says he divided his low-calorie diet into four meals to take advantage of the after-meal thermic effect. After all, digestion burns up calories. And before the blaze becomes a pile of embers, Dr. Miller recommends a brisk 20-minute walk. If done no later than 20 minutes after at least two meals a day, your postmeal heat production can be enhanced by up to 50 percent, he says. So, if your digestive processes normally burn 100 calories, a brisk walk for 20 minutes could increase that to 150. Do that after two meals each day and that's 36,500 calories a year—more than ten pounds of fat. "Exercise after meals burns calories more efficiently than any other exercise schedule," Dr. Miller says. "It's at this time that you're primed to increase your metabolic rate. So step on the gas. Take advantage of this maximum time."

Once you master two brisk walks a day, you might want to consider graduating into more aerobic exercises. Researchers at the University of New Hampshire found that an increase in aerobic capacity (your body's ability to use oxygen) significantly increases the number of calories you burn after a meal—even if you're *not* exercising at that particular time.

When they tested dietary-induced thermogenesis in a group of men and women, they discovered that those with greater aerobic capacity burned more calories after eating (or, in this case, drinking high- and low-calorie drinks). And the men (but not the women) were more likely to have a lower percentage of body fat. The best news, however, is that those not-terribly-fit people who improved their aerobic capacity by exercise were *also* able to stoke their after-meal blaze. One woman who increased her aerobic capacity by only 15 percent boosted her heat response by 110 percent (*European Journal of Applied Physiology,* vol. 50, no. 3, 1983).

Not everyone is going to be able to achieve the aerobic fitness of a well-conditioned athlete. Many of them have metabolisms that allow them to burn hundreds of calories while doing nothing more strenuous than watching television. Aerobic capacity can be increased only within limits because it largely depends on the number of muscle fibers you're born with. But, though you can't add muscle fibers, you can make the ones you have more effective through aerobic exercise.

Jogging, tennis, dancing—anything that gets your heart pumping and your muscles moving and forces your body to break down fat for energy—can increase your aerobic capacity. Aerobic exercise for 30 minutes three times a week will stimulate your metabolism so that you'll burn calories at a faster rate than usual for as long as 24 hours after exercise—*in addition* to the hundreds you'll be burning during the exercise. "Aerobic activity stimulates the metabolism better than any other factor," says Dr. Miller.

It does something else, too. It increases your muscle mass at the same time it reduces the amount of fat you're carrying. People who have a high ratio of muscle to fat have higher metabolic rates. They can eat more and not gain weight because they burn more, even when they're sleeping.

"The reason for this is that muscle tissue is metabolically more active than fat tissue," Dr. Miller says. "It takes more body energy for muscle to function. Fat is relatively inactive, while muscle cells are extremely active, even when you are resting. A muscle furnace is constantly burning food fuel at a rapid rate day after day."

So to review, exercise can boost your metabolism in at least three different ways in addition to the immediate calorie burnoff. First, when exercise follows a meal, it increases dietary thermogenesis—"roasting" calories that would otherwise be stored as fat. Second, regular aerobic exercise increases metabolism all day long—giving an extra boost after meals even if you're just reading a book. And third, by adding muscle, with its high metabolic rate, you're subtracting extra calories from your system every moment of the day.

But exercise and meal timing aren't the only factors that affect your metabolism. What you eat, even the temperature of your home, can either fan the fires or hose them down.

Eating to Lose

Eat more fruits, vegetables and whole grains, the complex carbohydrates. Avoid fats and simple carbohydrates (candy, soft drinks, desserts). Elliot Danforth, Jr., M.D., director of the clinical research center at the University of Vermont, says a return "to the diet of our ancestors" can have a significant impact on obesity. That means a diet that is about two-thirds complex carbohydrates and the rest protein and fat. Why? "There's a clear biochemical reason for this," says Dr. Danforth, who did many of the early studies on metabolism and obesity. "You expend only about 3 percent of your fat calories storing them as fat, but you expend 25 percent of your carbohydrate calories storing them as fat. The metabolic cost is far higher to store carbohydrates as fat. Any Iowa pig farmer will tell you. When you ask him how he gets his pigs so fat, he'll tell you it isn't by feeding them wheat, it's by feeding them fat."

Extremes of heat or cold increase your metabolism by as much as 10 percent, says Dr. Miller. Even a small deviation helps. Set your thermostat at 68°F in the winter and 79°F in the summer. You'll get used to the temperatures and your metabolism will get a boost.

Like most sensible weight-loss regimens, this is a lifetime proposition. Once you perk up your metabolism, it will be your ally. But you've got to keep it perked up through diet and exercise.

Open Your Lungs and Breathe Easy

How long could you live without food? Several weeks, perhaps? Without water? Maybe a few days? But without air, your survival would be measured in *minutes*. Though most of us take them totally for granted, our airways are literally our conduits to life. Yet for a growing number of Americans, keeping these vital lifeways open and functioning has become a real challenge.

An estimated 18 million people in this country find themselves gasping and wheezing from asthma, chronic bronchitis or emphysema. Together, these ailments are called chronic obstructive pulmonary disease, or COPD. And at a time when the incidence of heart disease is falling, the COPD rate is rising by 10 percent a year. In fact, lung disease has been called the nation's "most serious health threat" because of its increasing incidence.

Not all of the news about lung disease is bad, however. Pulmonary specialists say that it is easily within our power to prevent chronic bronchitis and emphysema—the two worst forms of COPD—and that more effective treatment of both may eventually be in reach.

The causes of chronic bronchitis (an inflammation of the larger airways) and emphysema (the blockage and destruction of the smaller airways) are no longer a mystery. Tobacco smoke is the number one cause of each of these illnesses, and most lung patients are veteran smokers. Even among coal miners and asbestos workers, those who develop lung disease are usually smokers.

"Without cigarettes, those two lung diseases would be uncommon," says Lawrence Martin, M.D., chief of the pulmonary division at Mt. Sinai Medical Center in Cleveland and author of *Breathe Easy: A Guide to Lung and Respiratory Disease for Patients and Their Families* (Prentice-Hall, 1984). "Even in industry, it is the smokers who have the most respiratory illnesses."

"Smoking may not be the whole story," adds Robert Sandhaus, M.D., Ph.D., of the National Jewish Hospital/National Asthma Center in Denver, "because there are a few people who smoke for 60 years and don't get sick. But for most lung patients, cigarette smoking is the common link."

Breath-Building Exercises

If smoking is the common link among those who develop lung disease, then exercise is one of the links among those who fight back most successfully. Even though exercise may be the last thing an emphysema patient feels able to do, it must be done. The reason: Trained muscles need less oxygen than weak ones.

"Emphysema patients get so out of breath when they walk because their muscles are inefficient for their condition," Dr. Sandhaus explains. "When they do start exercising, they won't necessarily feel stronger, but they'll find that they aren't out of breath so often."

"Strong muscles require less oxygen because they're more efficient," agrees Pat Peabody, an R.N. who works with lung patients in Monterey, California. "A well-tuned car uses less gas, and well-tuned muscles use less oxygen."

"We advise our patients to walk—not jog—a mile every day," Dr. Martin adds, "and in the winter we ask them to walk in shopping malls."

Breathing exercises are just as important as leg exercises. One breathing exercise that might help would be to practice breathing deeply and letting the air out slowly. One technique is called belly breathing. The idea is to push the stomach out on the inhalations and then to suck it back in on the exhalations. This strengthens the diaphragm, which is the muscle that ideally should expand and contract the lungs.

Another technique is called pursed-lip breathing. Air has a tendency to be trapped in diseased lungs, and pursed-lip breathing helps people exhale more thoroughly. Janice Volk, a physical therapist at Monmouth Medical Center in New Jersey, says, "When you exhale, close your lips and breathe out as if you were blowing out a candle. Breathe out twice as long as you breathe in. This helps to keep the airways open longer to get rid of stale air."

Vitamins Advised

Nutrition also plays a major role in the treatment of chronic lung disease. In fact, it is becoming popular among some doctors who doubted its value in the past.

"We are using what is still an unproved theory, which is unusual for us," says Dr. Sandhaus. "We know that the oxidants in cigarette smoke are what damage the lungs. And we know that vitamin C and vitamin E are both antioxidants. That is why we are advising a minimum of 250 milligrams of vitamin C twice a day and 800 international units (I.U.) of vitamin E, also twice a day, for all of our emphysema patients." [*Editor's Note:* Dosages of vitamin E in excess of 1,200 I.U. daily should best be taken under a doctor's supervision.]

"We also stress nutrition," says Dr. Martin. "We ask our patients to eat regular meals if they can. Sometimes they can't eat a large meal because a full stomach can press against their diaphragm and make breathing harder. If that is the case, we tell them to eat several small meals instead."

There is also evidence that selenium deficiency weakens the repair mechanism that would normally counteract the damage done to the lungs by cigarette smoke. A recent study of emphysema patients at the University of Pittsburgh showed that vitamin C, vitamin E and selenium all help protect the lung tissue from oxidants (*Study on Synthesis of Pathology Research,* vol. 3, no. 1, 1984).

Drugs are a fact of life for many people with chronic lung disease. Asthma and chronic bronchitis sufferers need bronchodilators to open up their constricted air sacs. Without such drugs, many people would die. But medication often has pitfalls that patients should know about.

Some people, for example, unnecessarily resign themselves to the side effects of their medication. "A lot of people get the shakes and their appetite vanishes as a result of the drugs," says Mrs. Peabody. "But they don't tell their doctors. They just say to themselves, 'I must be getting older, that's all.'"

Dr. Martin emphasizes that each person must have the patience to find the medication and dosage that is right for them. There are hundreds of possible drug combinations and dosages, he says. He keeps in "constant contact by phone" with new patients, asking them what side effects they are or are not encountering.

Of all the drugs used for lung problems, the cortico-steroids are the most potent. When all else fails, the steroids are brought in to improve breathing. Physicians don't know exactly how steroids work, but they agree that this class of drugs is for short-term use only. Dr. Martin advises against using oral steroids for more than two weeks at a time.

Reversing the Irreversible

Another major issue in the pulmonary field is the question of reversibility. Among doctors, traditional wisdom dictates that asthma is treatable and reversible, that chronic bronchitis is treatable but not reversible, and that emphysema is neither treatable nor reversible.

But doctors are now revising their positions on reversibility. They've discovered that emphysema patients often suffer to some extent from asthma, and are therefore at least partially treatable.

"It's rare to find a case of pure emphysema," says Dr. Sandhaus. "There is usually a component of asthma or chronic bronchitis, which is treatable or reversible. We also have medications that reduce the mucus production that's characteristic of bronchitis, and that can lead to better breathing for every patient.

"Just because people have emphysema doesn't mean that they can't breathe better," he adds. "We are even finding out that the lungs might be able to repair the damage caused by emphysema" — though that lies in the future.

Dr. Martin doesn't give up either, even on those emphysema patients who have given up on themselves. "We try not to label people as having 'emphysema' or 'chronic bronchitis,' " he says. "We evaluate people individually. We start from scratch.

"We go for every bit of reversibility we can get. If we see someone who is breathing at only 40 percent of normal capacity, then we try to push them up to 60 percent. That can make then feel like a new person. That can make the difference between someone leading a normal life or not," Dr. Martin says.

Lung patients need that kind of morale boost, because depression is a constant hazard for them. "When you can't breathe, you become very alarmed," says Jean Taylor, a 62-year-old bronchitis sufferer in Monmouth County, New Jersey. "Some people become so frightened that they are unable to go on with their lives. So many people become invalids. But once you understand the disease and accept it — the more you become aware — then you can go on with your life."

The best way to avoid this predicament, of course, is to prevent lung damage in the first place. Not smoking is the single most important factor. But paying attention to the early warning signs of lung disease is also critical. The first indications of emphysema and bronchitis may appear years before a person reaches the severe stage of the disease, when it requires emergency care.

"I've asked people how long they've been coughing and they say, 'For years—but it's just a smoker's cough,'" Dr. Martin says. "But it isn't normal to cough up sputum every morning.

"Someone else might tell me that she hasn't been able to climb stairs for years. But she'll say, 'It doesn't bother me; I live in a ranch house.' A lot of people ignore the early signs of lung disease," Dr. Martin says.

"People often live with the symptoms of lung disease for 10 to 15 years before they seek medical help," adds Phyllis Krug, a New Jersey physical therapist. "They tell themselves, 'I'm just getting a little short of breath,' or 'I guess I'm getting old,' or 'It couldn't happen to me.' Sometimes they would rather not find out that they have emphysema. There's a tremendous amount of denial with lung disease."

Hopefully, as public awareness of lung disease grows, denial will give way to prevention so that someday no one will need to "starve" for want of something as freely available as air.

Preventing and Relieving Varicose Veins

Ask your doctor what you can do about varicose veins, and he might advise you to choose your parents wisely. A weak smile will pass your lips before he explains that the affliction is largely hereditary, and since the genetic cards have already been dealt, it's time for feeble wit and making the most of your pair of deuces.

"It's an inherited disease," says Robert Nabatoff, M.D., a clinical professor of vascular surgery at Mt. Sinai School of Medicine in New York City.

"There's really not much you can do to prevent varicose veins. There are 15-year-olds who have them and 80-year-olds who do not have any trace of them. If you're going to get them, you're going to get them."

Not quite so, says another authority. "We don't inherit varicose veins; we inherit a *tendency* to develop varicose veins," says Howard Baron, M.D., attending vascular surgeon at Cabrini Medical Center in New York City and author of *Varicose Veins: A Commonsense Approach to Their Management* (William Morrow and Co.). "That's an important distinction."

Indeed, since implicit in the distinction is the conclusion that varicose veins can be prevented. And whether it's a belief in genetic certainty or some other factor, much of the medical advice on varicose veins deals with treatment rather than prevention. But the truth is that you can do much to prevent the onset of varicose veins, even if you *are* genetically likely to get them.

And if you can prevent them for a little while, it follows that you may be able to prevent them for a long while, or perhaps forever.

Doctors say that exercise, diet and support hosiery are all ways to prevent this affliction, which affects one in four American women and one in ten American men.

More Than a Nuisance

Many of us today might think of varicose veins as simply a cosmetic problem, particularly troubling in the summer months when the legs are more exposed in shorts, swimwear and dresses. For some that's the case. For others, however, varicose veins cause fatigue, dull aches in the legs, swelling and sleep-inhibiting cramps. And in a small percentage of cases, complications set in that could be life-threatening, like phlebitis, the development of clots in the deeper veins, and ulceration.

"People who think of varicose veins as only a nuisance are severely underestimating the disease," Dr. Baron says.

A varicose vein is nothing more than a healthy vein gone awry. It didn't start as a varicose vein; it became one. Here's how:

The veins help to transport blood from the legs back to the heart and lungs, where the blood is cleansed of its impurities (carbon dioxide, mostly) and refueled with oxygen for another trip through the body.

The blood has a more difficult journey from the lower

extremities because it's fighting gravity. Fortunately, the leg muscles act like a second heart. As the muscles contract, blood is pumped through the veins. The veins in turn are equipped with valves that act like locks on a canal.

The valves allow the blood to flow upward, then snap shut to prevent backward seepage. When the valves are too weak to prevent this gravitational backward flow, blood begins to collect in the vein, stretching the vein wall out of shape and producing pain and the often-unsightly varicosity.

Almost all varicosities occur in the veins near the surface of the leg. Deeper veins are rarely affected because they have support from muscle and fat.

"We inherit a defect in the venous valve or we inherit a vein with a weak or absent wall," Dr. Baron says. "Then there must be an aggravating factor in our lifestyle for the problem to develop. If we avoid aggravating factors, the problem might be delayed or blunted, and it might not develop at all."

Aggravating Factors

The aggravating factors are severe obesity, constipation, standing for prolonged periods, sitting for prolonged periods with your legs crossed and lack of exercise. A common thread runs through all of these factors: They all place added pressure on the surface veins of the legs, increasing the likelihood that varicosities will develop and progress.

Constipation's effect might not be obvious. Because the diets of many Westerners lack sufficient fiber, we tend to suffer from constipation more than peoples of the so-called Third World who have fiber-rich diets. Even when we're not constipated, our stools tend to be hard and pelletlike and difficult to pass. Both constipation and straining at stool increase intra-abdominal pressure, which is transferred to the veins of the legs. Think of the body as a totem pole, with the veins of the lower legs and ankles being the ultimate recipient of pressure from above.

One researcher, in fact, has theorized that constipation and straining at stool are among the primary causes of varicose veins. Denis P. Burkitt, M.D., of St. Thomas Hospital Medical School in London, a world-renowned expert on fiber, drew his conclusions after observing tribesmen in Africa who have fiber-rich diets and an exceedingly low incidence of varicose veins.

"It's not only varicose veins. We Americans get other diseases that people with fiber-rich diets don't get, like cancer of the colon and rectum," says Victor Pellicano, M.D., an internist in Lewiston, New York. "In the Western world it's the price we pay for eating so much processed food."

In short, eat more vegetables, fruits and whole grains, and don't strain at stool.

Exercise, too, can head off varicose veins. The flip side, of course, is that lack of exercise exacerbates the problem. "We're a sitting society," Dr. Baron declares. "I'm sitting right now. . . with my legs crossed. From 3 to 18, kids do nothing but sit. They sit at school, they sit while they're doing their homework, they sit while they watch television.

"My advice is to walk, run, jog, anything to keep the leg muscles working. Don't sit still. Don't stand still."

Prolonged standing in one place and sitting (particularly with the legs crossed, since that further impedes circulation) allows blood to pool in the lower extremities. That puts added pressure on a weak valve and can further dilate a vein with a weak wall. Either will hasten the onset of varicose veins. Exercise keeps the body's "second heart," the muscles of the lower legs, contracting and the valves clicking.

The best exercise regimen is to do some activity more often, rather than a lot at one shot. This presents a problem for people who are sedentary at work or who are temporarily captive in a plane or a theater. Those people can simply press the balls of their feet to the floor to make the calf muscles contract and transport blood. Nothing more elaborate is necessary.

If you have a job that requires that you be on your feet— bartender, beautician, retail clerk—take an elevation break. That is, prop your legs up so that they are higher than your heart several times during the day to allow gravity to speed the blood to the heart.

Support Hosiery and Other Solutions

If your boss won't agree to the break, support hosiery could be the answer. "Support hosiery is very helpful," Dr.

Pellicano says. "Not only does it give comfort to those who already have varicose veins, it could delay the onset of the problem for many years."

Support hosiery exerts graduated pressure on the leg and facilitates blood flow, thus reducing pressure in the veins.

A few other tips:

● Stop reading on the toilet. The shape of the hard wood or plastic seat puts undue pressure on the abdominal veins, which, in turn, put pressure on the leg veins.

● Don't wear any tight garment, particularly calf-length boots, panty hose too snug at the groin, girdles, corsets or binding belts. All of these tend to constrict venous blood flow.

● Be sure your diet contains oranges, tangerines or other citrus fruits. They are a good source of bioflavonoids, which may delay the onset of varicose veins. Bioflavonoids may do that, according to Dr. Pellicano, by strengthening the vein wall, preventing dilation and allowing the valves to work more easily.

As a factor relating to varicose veins, pregnancy has not been mentioned as something to avoid, for obvious reasons. Pregnancy has been linked to varicosities, but it's not causal. Dr. Baron calls pregnancy an "accelerator." What pregnancy does is increase pressure on pelvic veins, much like straining at stool would do, thus obstructing the drainage of blood from the legs.

The pregnancy link has led to the belief that women suffer more from varicose veins than men do, and statistics would appear to substantiate that. But Dr. Nabatoff has an alternative explanation. "Varicose veins are largely a cosmetic thing," he says, "and when women notice them, they're quick to get them treated. Men often ignore the problem. There are plenty of men who have varicose veins. They just don't seek treatment."

The beauty of the recommendations made by the doctors cited here is that they might stop varicose veins from appearing or, if they have appeared already, the discomfort may be less acute.

Gloria Bayer knows what it's like to keep a constant vigil against the pain of varicose veins. "What's annoying," she says, "is having to be so conscious of it all the time."

When she says "all the time" to describe her state of awareness, she isn't exaggerating. When she gets out of bed in the morning, she begins walking immediately to head off the pain. As she showers she's careful not to stand still for too long, for it only takes a few minutes for the blood to pool and discomfort to begin. Throughout her workday, she exercises her leg muscles or elevates her legs at her desk. When she jogs she allows herself a five-minute cool-down period. And if she stands in line anywhere—at the bank, at the grocer's, at the theater—she does in-place exercises to keep the muscles working and the blood from collecting.

"The pain won't stop on its own," she says. "It'll only get worse if you continue to do what you're doing. In a way it's made me more active. I don't stand still much anymore."

Surgical Option

Gloria Bayer's attentiveness has kept her varicose vein problem from worsening. But if your condition has deteriorated to the point where the varicose veins are large and the pain is becoming more and more of a burden, you might want to consider having them removed.

"If you have varicose veins and they're not treated, you're ten times more likely to get phlebitis, clots and ulceration," Dr. Nabatoff says. "The veins that stick out are susceptible to trauma, irritation and bleeding at the ankle. Almost all ulceration occurs at the ankles." There are two options.

Surgical Removal ● This procedure is commonly called stripping. The varicose veins are tied off and removed. This procedure usually involves an overnight stay in the hospital and several days' rest. But once the vein is gone, so is the varicosity. The condition could possibly recur though, when smaller, previously little-used but diseased veins take over the job of circulating the blood.

The drawbacks to stripping? "Anytime you go under general anesthesia, there's a greater risk and sometimes there's bleeding that can't be controlled without going back in to tie it off," says James DeWeese, M.D., a cardiovascular surgeon at the University of Rochester Medical Center.

"The operation is a simple one for any competent vascular surgeon," Dr. Baron says. "And there's a 96 percent cure rate. That means that three years after the operation there is no reappearance of the varicosity in 96 percent of the cases."

Injection Therapy ● In a procedure done in the doctor's office, a chemical solution is injected into the affected vein, causing it to harden and wither away over a period of several months. This procedure works best on smaller varicose veins. "Large varicose veins with high backward pressure don't respond to injection therapy," Dr. Nabatoff says. "If you inject that type, they just recur. The heavy ones you have to tie and strip." With both procedures, the patient should be seen again on a yearly basis.

Dr. Baron feels that injection therapy can be dangerous. "What you're doing is forming a chemical phlebitis, and if you're unlucky the clot could extend and make its way into a large vein," he says. Frequently, there are pigment changes at the injection site that are permanent.

It should be clear that varicose veins are a complex problem. If a close family member has the affliction, you're at risk, but fortunately there's much you can do to prevent the condition. And even if you have varicose veins, preventive measures can help ease your discomfort.

Medical Facts to Help You Look Younger

It could be a scene right out of a cold cream commercial. You're at a high school class reunion, looking eagerly for a friend you haven't seen in 20 years. But when she approaches, you barely recognize her. Her hair and figure are fine, and she's as lively and funny as ever. But her face is lined and weathered. As you greet her, you can't help asking yourself: "Do I look that old, too?"

We judge people's age and health, and maybe even their sexual attractiveness or ability to do a job right, by what we see in their faces. That's why it's important to know what yours is saying about you. If it's making you look tired or older than you feel, more than simple vanity could be at stake. Having to look at a world-weary face in the mirror every morning could erode your self-confidence and change the way people treat you. If you're an older woman in business or you're looking for a mate, you could face outright discrimination or rejection, says Albert Kligman, M.D., Ph.D., professor of dermatology at the University of Pennsylvania Medical School and director of the Clinic for Aging Skin in Philadelphia.

"I think wrinkles are a major medical and psychological problem, far more serious than most doctors acknowledge," Dr. Kligman says. "They may not be a threat to life, but the anxieties they create can spoil life. I think there are good psychological and economic reasons for that anxiety, especially among women. One thing I *don't* tell them is that they have to accept their face the way it is. There are plenty of things women can do to smooth the wrinkles they have and to prevent more."

And plastic surgery isn't the only route, as we'll see.

Line by Line

First let's take a look at what happens as a face ages.

Most people show faint signs of aging by around age 30, says Gerald Imber, M.D., a plastic surgeon at the Institute for the Control of Facial Aging in New York City. Most often these signs are squint lines around the corners of the eyes or faint horizontal lines across the forehead. Like a leather glove, the skin becomes permanently creased into wrinkles in the areas where it's being worked into frequent expressions.

By age 40, wrinkles from other facial expressions have shown up—arcs running from the nose to the corners of the mouth and vertical lines between the eyebrows. By age 50, these wrinkles have become deeper. The skin on the cheeks and neck starts to loosen up and sag into jowls and "turkey neck."

By age 60, these features may be established. The muscles around the eyes may have weakened, allowing fat deposits to pop through and form bags under the eyes.

By age 70, wrinkles have formed everywhere. The skin is rougher in texture and has lost its uniform color. Ovals of deeper pigmentation—liver spots—dot the forehead and temples. The risk of melanoma, a potentially deadly skin cancer, is double what it was at age 30. And the risk of getting the usually treatable squamous, or basal cell, cancer is 60 times greater.

Both the tip of the nose and the earlobes have drooped about half an inch or more. The skin has redraped itself over the underlying bone structure so that prominent features, like a big nose, seem to stand out even more. But pleasing features also stand out.

"If you have good bone structure, you will appear to age better," Dr. Imber says. "Noticeable facial prominences like high cheekbones, forehead and chin maintain certain highlights so that when the light hits them, they stand out and give form to the face. This constantly maintains the look of youth and vitality." And people with a right angle between the jaw and neck will have less noticeable sagging of the skin beneath the jaw than those whose jaw and neck tend to meet in a curving line, Dr. Imber says.

These facial changes are mostly the result of damage in the supporting tissues lying beneath the paper-thin top layer of skin. This tissue, known as the dermis, contains water, fat and spindly, star-shaped cells called fibroblasts. These cells help produce a network of fibers that weave through the dermis to support the skin. The two most important fibers are collagen and elastin. Together, they give firmness and elasticity to the skin, making it bounce back after it's stretched into a smile or a scowl.

But as we age, the dermis retains less water and fat, so the skin doesn't look as firm and plump. Oil-producing cells slow their production, so the skin gets drier. The cell renewal rate slows, especially in women past menopause. New cells don't develop as quickly and old ones stay longer on the surface of the skin. Fibroblast cells produce fewer supporting fibers, and those that are produced have less resiliency than in young skin. The skin receives less oxygen and nutrients as tiny capillaries beneath it close off.

All this may seem nasty and inevitable and something we're better off not knowing about at all. But the fact is that even though dermatologists and plastic surgeons talk about these skin changes as part of the aging process, aging alone does *not* cause these changes. How fast our faces age and, indeed, whether they ever show all these changes depends on a number of factors—most of which are within our control.

The only factor we can't control is genetics. People with dark, thick, oily skin get the fewest wrinkles, mainly because that heavily pigmented outer layer protects the dermis from the harmful effects of sunlight. Fair-skinned redheads and blonds, who usually burn rather than tan, are most wrinkle prone.

The other factors—sun protection, exercise, not smoking, eating well and managing the stress in our lives—are all within our control.

Be a Shady Character

Sure, you've heard it all before. Sunlight hurts your skin. But do you really know just how much of a hazard it is? Many dermatologists think the sun is the *number one* cause of wrinkling, pigment changes and skin cancer.

"It's sunlight that produces what most people think of as aging skin," Dr. Kligman says. "I always show women the underside of their breast or upper arm, areas that are seldom exposed to the sun. That's the way the skin on their faces would look if it had been protected—smooth, firm, umblemished."

The good news is that even if you've overdone the sun in the past, it's never too late to see improvement by limiting your exposure now.

"If you stay in the shade or use a sunscreen, you will see reversal of many of the changes in your skin," Dr. Kligman says. "It won't become young skin again. The major changes—wrinkles, bags, sags—are going to stay. But the connective tissues underneath the top layer of the skin, the dermis, will definitely improve. The fibroblasts have a chance to make new collagen. Precancerous lesions simply disappear. After about two or three years of not being in the sun, you'll have what looks like a light peel, where a few upper layers of the skin have been removed, leaving the skin smoother looking."

Wear a sunscreen any time you're going to be outside for more than a few minutes, dermatologists recommend. The higher the sun protection factor (SPF), the better. Find a product that feels good on your skin so you'll use it regularly. If your skin seems to be sensitive to a sunscreen, try different brands until you find one your skin can tolerate. Use a water-proof brand if you're swimming or sweating.

Jog Those Wrinkles Away

Know how a good brisk workout brings a healthy glow to your cheeks? Well, that blush isn't just pretty. It's a sign that the exercise is flushing your skin with blood. And the result is good news for wrinkle watchers, says James White, Ph.D., an exercise physiologist at the University of California, San Diego, and author of *Jump for Joy* (Arco Publishing, 1984), a book of exercise programs for people concerned about their skin or recovering from plastic surgery.

Finnish researchers, for example, found that middle-aged athletes had skin that was denser, thicker and stronger than that of a matched group of sedentary people. The elastic quality that allows the skin to spring back to its original shape after being stretched was also significantly better in the athletes.

The cells in the base layer of the skin, where skin cells are formed, actually become more active with exercise, Dr. White says. More of the chemical substances that are used to produce the elastic fibers can be found in the cells of people who exercise.

In his own research, Dr. White used three-dimensional photographs to measure the number, depth, width and distribution of wrinkles in groups of women. He found that those who either worked out indoors on a minitrampoline or ran outdoors while using a sunblock, both for 30 to 40 minutes a day, had fewer wrinkles than nonexercisers. And the exercise group had an added bonus—the bags under their eyes vanished.

"I'm more than sure that exercise can increase the elasticity of the skin and improve its appearance, even in older people," Dr. White says. But, he cautions, use a sunblock faithfully when exercising outdoors, and protect your face from wind and cold. "Wear a neoprene face mask when it's really cold," he says. And if you swim regularly for exercise, apply a good moisturizer first to keep chlorine from being absorbed into your skin.

Puff on This

Ask a plastic surgeon to pick out the smokers in a crowd and he'll easily oblige you. "You absolutely can see a difference between the faces of smokers and nonsmokers," Dr. Imber says. "All women who smoke get vertical lines in their upper lips from drawing on the cigarette." And they also get more wrinkles, and deeper wrinkles, all over their faces, because nicotine constricts the tiny capillaries that nourish the skin.

And because smoking interferes with the healing process, it occasionally causes dangerously bad results following cosmetic surgery to smooth out those wrinkles, reports Thomas Rees, M.D., a plastic surgeon affiliated with the Manhattan Eye, Ear and Throat Hospital in New York City. Eighty percent of patients who had problems recovering from their facelifts smoked more than a pack a day. Thick layers of their skin died and fell off, resulting in larger scars and longer healing time.

Eat Right for Healthy Skin

Good nutrition is important for healthy, disease-free skin that's less likely to crack, peel or dry out. And healthy skin is less likely to show wear and tear, Dr. Imber says.

Skin problems are sometimes the first signal of a vitamin deficiency. Some B-complex deficiencies—of thiamine, riboflavin, biotin—cause scaling and redness, especially around the mouth and nose.

Zinc deficiencies can cause similar conditions. Both zinc and vitamin C are important in the production of collagen, the skin's support tissue.

Vitamin A is also especially important for healthy, normal growth of skin cells. Synthetic forms of vitamin A have been used to help treat cancerous and precancerous skin growths, and to treat both acne and wrinkles. In all cases it increases the cell renewal rate, normalizes cell growth, and stimulates blood flow and collagen formation, Dr. Kligman says.

Some of the antioxidant vitamins—A, C and E—seem to reduce the sun's damage to the skin. But whether taking them over a lifetime will make you less wrinkled is yet to be seen.

Give Yourself a Break

Again and again, dermatologists have seen the connection between stress and all kinds of skin diseases—an acne flare-up just before an exam, severe eczema during a divorce. There's no doubt our emotions can play havoc with our skin, but whether stress and worry can cause wrinkles is something that has yet to be verified, says Roland S. Medansky, M.D., an Illinois dermatologist.

"Compared to sun exposure and genes, I'd say stress plays a small part in aging skin," Dr. Medansky says. "But there's no question that it can cause skin to appear to age. All you have to do is look at the face of any president when he goes into office and when he comes out four years later. You might see double or triple that number of extra years on his face." Sometimes, surprisingly, that damage might tend to reverse itself later, as ex-presidents relax and enjoy their retirement. "Remember how pasty and lined Jimmy Carter looked when he left office?" one dermatologist asks. "Well, he looks a heck of a lot better now."

It's true we all eventually face the forces of time and gravity. "Most people can accept normal signs of aging," Dr. Imber says. "It's when the aging becomes accelerated or unsightly that it disturbs them." Avoid that by taking care of your face now, no matter what your age.

New Dimensions in Self-Care

What an Irregular Heartbeat Means

There you are, sitting down with a mug of coffee in the tranquillity of your own kitchen, when your heart races as if you'd just run up a flight of stairs. Or, sleeping on your left side, you're suddenly awakened by the pounding of your heart. Or, for no reason at all, you feel as if butterflies are fluttering where your heart should be. When this happens, it's scary enough to make you consider an immediate trip to the cardiologist.

Sometimes these arrhythmias, as they're called, do mean that something is wrong with the heart. Ventricular fibrillation, in which the heart beats randomly and recklessly, can lead to death. Certain kinds of bradycardia or tachycardia, which means the pulse is too slow or too fast, may mean that there is some underlying ailment.

But more often than not, temporary arrhythmias aren't cause for mental heartache. "Mild arrhythmias are the most common reason for referral to a cardiologist," one doctor told us, and others say that occasional mild arrhythmias "no more augur sudden death than a sneeze portends pneumonia." In fact, healthy people whose hearts *never* miss a beat are very much in the minority.

A significant advance in cardiology in recent years has

been the discovery that arrhythimias are common among normal, healthy people. Irregularities once thought to be life-threatening—fast pulse, ventricular ectopic beats (irregular beats) and even some types of heart block (a failure in the flow of electric impulses across the heart muscle)—happen to, but seem not to bother, people who are otherwise in good health.

In England not long ago, researchers set out to discover "the rhythm of the normal human heart," studying the electrocardiograms of 86 healthy people who had no trace of heart disease. To the scientists' surprise, most of the study group possessed a rhythm disturbance of some kind. The normal, in other words, was abnormal. To explain why these people seemed to do just fine even with arrhythmias, the researchers said, "Perhaps these disturbances may well be tolerated by a normal heart" (*Lancet,* September 4, 1976).

Others have agreed with them. "When ventricular ectopic beats occur in someone who has heart irregularities, they can generate a lethal disturbance," says Bart Gershen, M.D., "but in a healthy person, this arrhythmia might have no effects at all."

Indeed, even the healthiest people suffer arrhythmias. Dr. Gershen surveyed 50 healthy medical students at Holy Cross Hospital in Silver Spring, Maryland, and found that at least half showed skipped beats, palpitations or pounding in their chests, while their pulses at times soared as high as 180 and dropped as low as 37 beats per minute. Other cardiologists have found that harmless arrhythmias commonly show up in superfit distance runners, even while they run (*American Heart Journal,* October, 1982).

Arrhythmia and Age

It is also entirely normal, apparently, for arrhythmias to become more frequent as we get older. Even the elderly shouldn't become alarmed just because a few mild ventricular arrhythmias show up on their electrocardiograms. A survey of 106 active people over age 75 a few years ago showed that most of them had signs such as irregular beats or racing pulse, but the symptoms didn't cramp their lifestyle. In fact, among those 106 relatively healthy elderly persons, only 24 (23 percent) could boast of a "normal" heart rate for 24 hours straight (*American Heart Journal,* May, 1980).

Of course, cardiac arrhythmias are sometimes an indication that something has gone awry with the heart. This "something" could be anything from advanced heart disease to nothing more serious than a reaction to strong coffee.

Ventricular arrhythmias, for instance, often accompany a heart attack, appearing at the time of the attack and in the weeks that follow. It used to be gospel that arrhythmias following a heart attack could trigger a second attack. For that reason, doctors often plied their heart patients with antiarrhythmia drugs. But studies have shown that those arrhythmias are an effect rather than a cause of heart attack and may not require medication (*British Medical Journal,* September 1, 1979).

Similarly, atrial fibrillation, in which the heart may have an irregular rhythm, is associated with diabetes, and it greatly increases the chance of a fatal heart attack. But there's a more positive note: Atrial fibrillation is much less dangerous when it strikes someone with a fairly healthy heart (*New England Journal of Medicine,* April 29, 1982).

On the other hand, arrhythmias may not indicate a heart attack at all. They might be a symptom of magnesium deficiency.

Anyone who uses diuretic medication to control high blood pressure is a candidate for magnesium deficiency. Diuretics drain the body of magnesium, and they are among the most commonly prescribed types of drugs in America.

But those not on diuretics are also vulnerable. The average magnesium intake by Americans in 1900 was 475 milligrams a day. Today, however, the average daily intake is only 245 milligrams--well below the 300 to 350 milligrams a day recommended by the National Academy of Sciences.

"Any patient who is on diuretic therapy and has irregularities in the heart rhythm should be checked for serum magnesium levels," says Eugene Coodley, M.D., of the Veterans Administration Medical Center in Long Beach, California. "If they are low, they should be brought up with magnesium sulfate."

It should come as little surprise that magnesium is essential for a regular pulse. On a cellular level, a magnesium-dependent enzyme helps generate the energy that gives each heartbeat its oomph, and there have been cases in which people with life-threatening arrhythmias have recovered their natural rhythm with no other treatment than magnesium supplementation (*Acta Medica Scandinavica,* vol. 212, 1982).

Caffeine has been implicated as a dietary inducer of arrhythmia. Americans consume about 2.2 billion pounds of coffee a year, and the caffeine in that coffee disturbs the pulse possibly in the same way that it creates alertness and insomnia—by triggering the release of adrenaline. People with existing heart problems are especially vulnerable to caffeine, and for that reason most cardiac care units allow only decaffeinated beverages as a matter of policy (*New England Journal of Medicine,* April 7, 1983).

Coffee-induced arrhythmias, in fact, can be frightening, and they send many anxious people in search of a cardiologist. "We see a number of people who developed palpitations after their morning coffee," says Carl V. Leier, M.D., of Ohio State University. "Some people are more sensitive than others, and the phenomenon isn't universal," he says, "but about half of the people we see with arrhythmias also are coffee drinkers. If you have an arrhythmia and drink a lot of coffee, our advice would be to cut down."

Feelings the Heart Feels

Emotional stress can also raise the body's adrenaline levels and increase the likelihood of arrhythmias. The same high-stress life agenda that gives heart attacks to driven executives often gives them arrhythmias as well. Researchers at Harvard School of Public Health say that "psychological stress profoundly lowers the cardiac threshold for ventricular fibrillation"—the arrhythmia that causes sudden death.

Almost any kind of stress seems to do. Studies with animals have shown that such things as offering and denying food and mild physical restraint in unfamiliar surroundings may cause arrhythmia. In humans, feelings of abandonment, depression and alienation and even violent dreams are thought to cause arrhythmia.

Acute anger, researchers think, disrupts heart rhythms the most. Anger releases body chemicals that may constrict the arteries that supply the heart itself with blood (*Annual Reviews in Physiology,* 1984).

There is also a link between alcohol, cigarettes and cardiac arrhythmias, but doctors aren't sure how strong it is. In one of the studies mentioned here, British researchers found no obvious relationship between smoking and the type or number of arrhythmias in people over age 75. Another study has shown that, in a group of men and women in good health, smokers had faster but not less regular heart rates.

But nicotine, like anger, unleashes adrenaline and "cigarette smoking has been shown to lower the threshold for ventricular fibrillation during a heart attack." Dr. Coodley urges his heart patients to "reduce all coffee and alcohol and eliminate tobacco" because all "are capable of initiating arrhythmias."

As for alcohol, this oft-abused substance is known to be responsible for a syndrome called holiday heart. Every year between Christmas Eve and New Year's Day, apparently, hospital emergency rooms are frequented by people who develop severe arrhythmias as a result of alcoholic binges. In many cases, the specific arrhythmia is atrial fibrillation. It usually subsides when the alcohol wears off.

Many doctors believe that holiday heart occurs only among alcoholics or those with a long history of immoderate drinking. But Dr. Gershen says, "Any time someone overdrinks, there's the possibility of an irregular heartbeat. Alcohol is a potential toxin to the heart, and you don't have to be an alcoholic to be affected by it."

Almost any stimulant can adversely affect the heart, Dr. Gershen says, even the low-grade stimulants that are found in over-the-counter drugs. "A lot of the cold remedies that are available without a prescription contain ingredients that affect the heart," he says. "Most of them contain cardiac stimulants and you'll see if you read the package that they shouldn't be taken by people with high blood pressure.

"Even people without heart disease can develop rhythm disturbances from these drugs," he adds, "and they definitely can scare people" who might experience sudden palpitations without knowing why.

If an arrhythmia doesn't respond to changes in diet or lifestyle, a cardiologist may prescribe medication. These medications sometimes backfire and aggravate the very problem they are meant to solve, however. "Drugs are given to prevent a simple arrhythmia from developing into a more serious one," says Arthur Selzer, M.D., a San Francisco cardiologist. "But once in a while they can have the opposite effect," Other doctors have pointed out that "all the antiarrhythmic drugs that we have studied may aggravate arrhythmias."

Pacemakers are an option for those with a specific kind of arrhythmia called heart block, in which the heart's own electrical circuitry fails. Pacemakers are implanted in a heart patient's body and they can run for several years. They're intended mainly for the heart patient who suffers frequent fainting spells. Some doctors feel that pacemakers are too often installed unnecessarily. Dr. Selzer points out that pacemakers are used twice as often in the United States as they are in Europe, and that anyone who hasn't fainted and feels generally healthy should get a second opinion before accepting a pacemaker.

Can the average person participate in relieving his or her own arrhythmia? Yes, says Dr. Gershen. The first step is to identify it. Sudden flushing is sometimes a sign of arrhythmia. So is fatigue, especially if it's accompanied by difficulty with sleeping on the left side, where the heart is pressed between your chest and the mattress. And there are other signs.

"If someone is constantly aware of his or her heart, and if the rhythm disturbances occur frequently—several times a week—or if they last a long time, for several hours or so, then the person should probably see a doctor," Dr. Gershen says.

The next step might be to increase your intake of magnesium-rich foods, such as whole grains, dark green vegetables and beans. Giving up coffee and cigarettes, if you use them, is another tactic. Avoiding alcohol would probably be a good idea. And an attempt to resolve emotional stress may also help.

But the most important strategy is the prevention of heart

disease in the first place. The experts agree that cardiac arrhythmias are more common among heart disease sufferers and that, when they occur, arrhythmias are more likely to damage a frail heart than a strong one. The way to keep the heart strong is to adopt a healthy, low-fat, high-fiber diet, a regimen of regular exercise and a relaxed, positive attitude. That is also the best way to prevent cardiac arrhythmias.

Safe Home Remedies for Aches and Pains

Home-remedy painkillers?

Sure, Dad would have said, "Which do you want, whiskey or brandy?"

We've learned a lot since then. We know there are "home remedies" or natural treatments for pain that really make sense—without leaving you senseless.

They work like any other painkiller, giving you instant comfort rather than permanent cure. In the long run, you'll probably have to undertake an exercise program to make your aching back fit again and deal with the stress that brought on your headache in the first place. But you can do that once today's pain is gone.

A cautionary note: If pain is your enemy, consider it a friendly one. It's your body's way of telling you something is wrong. You don't want to mask the causes of pain. If you have a serious condition or if pain persists, see a physician. Only minor aches and pains should be treated at home.

Headache

● If your face feels tight, your nose is full, and your headache seems to be enveloping your face as well, you probably have a sinus headache. Steam or moist heat may help. If you can't get to a steam bath, make your own. Sit in the bathroom with the shower running hot and hard. Or try a warm pack across the eyes and cheekbones. Take a fluffy, thick washcloth and soak it in warm water. After you wring it out, apply it to the area that hurts. When it cools off, warm it up and reapply for about ten minutes. A steam vaporizer can be of inestimable value when a sinus headache hits.

● According to migraine expert Seymour Diamond, M.D., you can run away from a headache. Running, at least in theory, increases the production of endorphins, the body's natural painkillers. Dr. Diamond, executive director of the National Migraine Foundation and director of the Diamond Headache Clinic in Chicago, thinks these natural painkillers may be responsible for the relief migraine sufferers experience after jogging. For people who find running relaxing, he says, it could also relieve a muscle tension headache.

● About 90 percent of all headaches are so-called mechanical headaches, says Lionel A. Walpin, M.D., of the Walpin Physical Medicine Institute in Los Angeles. Mechanical headaches are those related to posture and its effects on muscles, ligaments and joints, says the physician and teacher. Relief may be as simple as changing the way you sleep, breathe or hold your tongue.

The advice from Dr. Walpin:

● Don't sleep on your stomach. When you do, your head is turned to one side, which can put too much pressure on the side of the jaw and upper neck, causing a headache. Dr. Walpin has even co-developed a pillow—called the WalPilO—a four-in-one cervical pillow that, among other things, discourages you from sleeping in that awkward stomach position and allows your muscles to relax, leading to more restful sleep.

● Breathe through your nose, not your mouth. Not only will you draw more air into your lungs, you'll hold your head and shoulders in a better posture in relation to your body. "You shouldn't use your neck and upper chest to breathe," says Dr. Walpin. "They're not designed for that. If you do, they'll become sore and refer pain to your head and shoulders."

• Hold your tongue lightly on the roof of your mouth, resting on the ridges of the upper palate and just behind your upper teeth. Why? If it rests in the wrong place in your mouth, this tiny muscle can exert enough force to cause head and neck misalignment, which can lead to headaches and stiff necks. To make sure it's in the right place, says Dr. Walpin, say "Boston" and keep your jaw as it is, with your tongue just behind but not touching the upper teeth. If it feels natural, you've got it.

Facial Pain

● Look for a mechanical cause. Do you wear sunglasses? A researcher at the University of Arizona College of Medicine found that three young women who had complained of numbness, burning and pain beneath their eyes had only one thing in common: They had all begun wearing sunglasses recently. He theorized that the sunglasses caused the problem because they're bigger and can irritate the facial nerve.

● Try tryptophan. Researchers at Temple University in Philadelphia found that three grams of tryptophan administered in conjunction with a high-carbohydrate, low-fat and low-protein diet relieved facial pain and increased pain tolerance among 30 chronic pain patients. Tryptophan is an amino acid that is a precursor of serotonin, a neurotransmitter in the brain that increases the effectiveness of the body's endorphins.

Toothache

● At McGill University in Montreal, scientists discovered they could relieve toothaches with an ice massage—but not by massaging anywhere near the teeth. They treated patients suffering from acute dental pain by massaging the web between the thumb and index finger of the hand on the same side as the dental pain. Ice massage decreased the intensity of the dental pain by half in most of the patients (*Canadian Medical Association Journal,* January 26, 1980).

Neck Pain

● If your neck aches in the morning, the culprit may be your sleeping habits, says James Fries, M.D., author of *Arthritis: A Comprehensive Guide* (Addison-Wesley, 1979) and coauthor of *Take Care of Yourself* (Addison-Wesley, 1981). Sleep on a firm mattress and throw away your pillow. For the pain, try heat: a nice hot shower, hot compresses or a heating pad. To give your neck support, take a bath towel, fold it lengthwise so it's about four inches wide and wrap your neck with it, securing it with a safety pin or tape. This, says Dr. Fries, will clear up "nearly half of all neck pain problems" by simply supporting the neck and reminding you not to turn too quickly or too far.

Shoulder Pain

● Usually this common pain comes from the soft tissues near the joint and not from the bones or joints themselves, says Dr. Fries. Gentle heat usually helps (though sometimes so does a cold pack), followed by exercises to help maintain mobility in the joint.

● A good pain-relieving shoulder exercise is the pendulum swing: Lean over so your arm hangs like a pendulum and swing it around in ever-increasing circles.

● To ease shoulder pain, it might also help to improve your posture. The shoulder is anatomically susceptible to fatigue. Try to relax, not tense, your neck and upper back muscles when you're under stress.

Tennis Elbow

● Needless to say, you're probably going to have to improve your technique and follow a few other rules laid down by New York physical therapist Eileen Shepherd: Don't buy a prestrung racket (they're too tight); use a two-handed backhand; avoid frequent change from slow clay to faster asphalt (or vice versa); keep your elbow bent and keep your eye on the ball. For the immediate pain, physicians recommend heat and range-of-motion exercises as your best bet.

Side Stitches

● You're out for a short run when suddenly there's a painful catch just below your ribcage. It makes you stop and, probably instinctively, you do exactly what you're supposed to do: Breathe it away. You change your breathing pattern from deep, rhythmic breathing to shallow, quick breathing or vice versa. Breathing from your diaphragm should make you less susceptible to this minor ache.

Back Pain

● An estimated seven million people are treated for back pain on any given day. In fact, it's been calculated that 80 percent of us will have a bout with backache at some time in our lives. The causes of back pain are legion, as are the cures. You may have to try several, or a combination, before you find a remedy for yourself. What you don't want to do is rely on muscle relaxants and painkillers, says Dr. Fries. They may get you moving around, but you're also likely to reinjure your back when the pain is masked. Therefore, medication is best used when accompanied by the first rule of back care: rest.

● If it's an injury that's laying your back low, don't reach for the comfort of a heating pad, as most people do, says James J. Irrgang, a registered physical therapist and director of the Center for Sports Medicine at the National Hospital for Orthopedics and Rehabilitation in Arlington, Virginia. For trauma, reach for ice. "It helps reduce inflammation and eliminate pain, and prevents much of the swelling from occurring," he says. "Heat can make all those things—inflammation, pain and swelling—much worse, especially right after the injury." An ice "popsicle" applied to the sore area for 15 minutes every four to six hours can effectively anesthetize the muscle spasm that accompanies back injuries such as muscle strain.

To make your ice pop, freeze a paper cup filled with water and then tear off the upper half. Peel the remainder as the ice melts.

● For the days following an injury or if your back problem is limited to pain and stiffness, especially on awakening, heat is your answer. A hot bath or shower, a heating pad, a hot-water bottle, or even hot, wet towels help. "Watch an old rheumatic dog and see how it searches out the sunniest part of the yard to warm its bones," says David Imrie, M.D., author of *Goodbye Backache* (Arco Publishing, 1983). So learn a new trick from an old dog.

● The worst enemy of your back may be your mattress. Many back sufferers find a nice firm mattress prevents the pain and stiffness that comes with morning. Others prefer a waterbed. A ¾-inch-thick piece of plywood under the mattress is a do-it-yourself mattress firmer.

● How you sleep is just as important as what you sleep on. The key to good sleeping habits is your knees, says C. David Tollison, Ph.D., author of *Managing Chronic Pain: A Patient's Guide* (Sterling Publishing Co., 1982). By bending your knees, you unlock your spine into a neutral position, which relieves muscle and ligament stress. That's why many backache sufferers prefer the fetal position: lying on the side with the hips and knees bent toward the chest and the head on the pillow. A second pillow between the knees will support the upper leg so circulation in the lower leg isn't blocked and will also prevent the lower back from twisting. If you sleep on your back, put a pillow under your knees to eliminate the swayback position you create when you lie flat on your back with your knees straight.

● Get rid of your fluffy foam-rubber pillow, which can lead to back and neck stiffness.

● Change positions frequently, not only while you're sleeping but while you're working, too. Remaining in one place too long can turn your sore muscles to stone. You can literally move away your pain.

● Correct your posture. Many backache problems can be prevented—and pain lessened—if you learn how to sit, stand and move properly. But, warns Dr. Walpin, who is currently writing a book on posture, don't assume the exaggerated military posture drilled into you at school. "Who can walk around like that?" he says. Your body, especially the upper chest and back, should be flexible, not stiff and at attention. Your head should be straight, with your chin and stomach slightly tucked in and your buttocks tucked slightly under. Then your spine will be at its natural curve.

● If you stand for long periods, put one foot on a stool, alternating every few minutes, says Dr. Tollison. "Prolonged standing fatigues the hip muscles and slowly pulls the pelvis forward." This causes a strain on the lower back muscles, which is relieved by lifting the foot slightly to return the spine to its natural curve.

● Sitting may be more stressful to your back than standing, since you lose the support of the pelvis when you sit down. If you have a bad back, don't cross your legs! It tilts the pelvis too far forward.

● Try to sit with your knees level with or slightly higher than your hips. Evelyn Rossky, an occupational therapist at Moss Rehabilitation Hospital in Philadelphia, advises her patients who must sit for long periods to get a two-inch-thick slab of Styrofoam to place under their feet as a footrest.

● Two of the best-selling items at Boston's The Back Store are the Balans chair, which tilts slightly forward to relieve pressure from the lower back and transfer weight to the midthigh, and a car seat cushion that adjusts the spine to a more comfortable angle. Dr. Walpin has helped develop a contoured seat cushion (called "Bottoms Up" pelvic spinal posture aid) that supports the pelvis while limiting the harmful effects of gravity on the spine and pelvis. Those are just a few of the products available to take a load off your back.

● Some women find their backaches disappear miraculously when they take off their shoes. Others may not feel immediate pain when they wear high heels, but over a period of time, Dr. Walpin warns, high heels can cause slow, subtle damage to the back. "It's okay to wear shoes with heels up to an inch and a half," says Dr. Walpin.

● If you feel a back twinge coming on, lie on the floor with your head and buttocks supported by pillows and your legs resting on a chair. The trunk of your body should be moved as close to the chair as possible. This position will probably make you feel so good "you may find yourself becoming addicted to it," says Dr. Imrie.

● Massage is nice anytime, but it's especially good when backache plagues your days and nights. Massage is a good way to work out a muscle spasm. It helps increase blood flow to the painful area and makes it relax.

● Stretch! Find yourself some good stretching exercises—even imitate a cat if you have to. Stretching enhances the flexibility of your back muscles and can give you momentary relief as well.

Muscle and Joint Aches

● Rest and exercise. It's as simple as that. You need to rest and relax a pained muscle or joint to ease the pain, and you need to exercise to avoid stiffness and more pain. A regimen of warm baths, massages and stretching exercises is good, according to Dr. Fries. He also recommends sponge-soled shoes for those who work on hard floors.

● If you do a lot of reading or needlework, try doing them with a fat, lightweight pillow across your lap, suggests Evelyn Rossky. Not only will it support the weight of your arms, it will invite better posture and eliminate the chin-on-chest position.

● Wrap foam on the handles of tools you use often—even pens and pencils—to take the strain out of gripping, says Ms. Rossky. You can even use the foam cylinder from a curler.

Knee Pain

● Try "Baggie therapy." That's the name coined by a group of doctors at a Philadelphia hospital who found that bags of ice placed on arthritic knees for 20 minutes gave sufferers more movement and strength and helped them sleep better and take less pain medication.

Leg Cramps

● They sneak up on you at night, an agonizing cramp in your leg (or foot) that seems to be ripping your muscle to shreds. Don't draw up your leg—stretch it. Get up and walk around, or massage or knead it like a lump of dough until it relaxes. A warm cloth also may help soften and calm the tensed muscle.

Menstrual Cramps

From the Federation of Feminist Women's Health Centers come these tips:

● Relax from head to toe. Lie back, rest your head on a pillow and elevate your legs over another. Concentrate on relaxing each set of muscles successively. Since the uterus is a muscle, you should find some relief from painful cramping.

● Try a direct uterine massage. Press on the spot just above the pubic hairline where the uterus is located and massage gently.

● Have someone apply pressure to your lower back.

● Do the cobra exercise: Lie flat on the floor, gradually raising your head and chest without using your arms until your upper body is off the floor. Now, using your arms, raise your torso so your back is arched. Repeat several times until the lower back muscles relax.

Foot Pains

● For corns, that old standby moleskin will do just fine, according to Timothy Shea, D.P.M., coauthor of *The Over*

Easy Foot Care Book (Scott, Foresman and Co., 1984). Cut plain moleskin into strips and place them on the corns to reduce the friction between your toes and shoes.

● Heal hard, ugly calluses by soaking your feet for 15 minutes in warm water and applying moisturizer two or three times a day. Once they're soft, says Dr. Shea, rub them with a pumice stone or another abrasive.

● For fallen arches, you should exercise, advises the podiatrist. Curl your toes, stretch your feet and rotate them to avoid the pain that radiates into your lower back.

● Massage sore feet with a foot roller or an empty soda bottle, gently rolling it back and forth with each foot several times a day.

● If your feet are stiff but not swollen, soak them in warm water for 15 minutes once or twice a day. If you have swelling, follow a 5-minute warm-water soak with 2 minutes in cool water, then repeat. This should be done twice a day, says Dr. Shea.

Burns

● Cold water usually relieves the pain of a minor burn. So does aloe vera. Use the fresh mucilaginous juice, applied directly from the plant leaf. Reapply as needed.

Have a Happy Tummy

Surely you've talked to your stomach. "Just one more bite." Or, "I can't believe we ate the whole thing."

And perhaps it's talked back. "Blurp. Blop. Gurgle. What do you mean, *we?*"

Maybe you've been downright rude to each other.

"I've never been so embarrassed in my life, and it's all your fault!"

"Oh, yeah? Well, if you hadn't devoured all those spare-ribs. . .and what was the marshmallow goop you ate? Maybe if you'd been a little more discriminating last night you wouldn't need to find fault today! (Snicker, snicker.)"

We all have occasional upsets from overeating, the flu or a food that just doesn't meet our stomach's high standards. The cramps, bloating, nausea or diarrhea may stay for a day or two, then disappear. Chances are we won't see a doctor unless the pain becomes severe or we're sick longer than three days. And in fact, there's not much to do except rest, eat plain, simple foods and watch "Little House on the Prairie."

Symptoms are the digestive tract's way of signaling how it's working. Learning to read its messages is important, both for self-care and to know when to see a doctor. Let's work our way through the digestive tract, looking at the messages organs send when there's trouble brewing.

Heartburn

Heartburn, due to esophageal reflux, is a pain or burning behind the breastbone, usually radiating upward into the chest. It can happen as soon as you start eating or any time soon after a meal. It's caused by the escape of stomach contents through the lower esophageal valve into the esophagus.

"The pain is worse when you lie down, and at night can cause coughing if some of the stomach contents are inhaled into the lungs," says Denis McCarthy, M.D., professor of medicine at the University of New Mexico and chief of gastroenterology at the Veterans Administration Hospital in Albuquerque.

Almost everyone has occasional heartburn, usually from too much food combined with smoking and bad posture, Dr. McCarthy says. But some people have symptoms every day, and for them the pain can be intense. Luckily, the following measures can eliminate most cases of heartburn, he says.

● Eat smaller, more frequent meals, and don't eat for at least three hours before bed.

● Don't smoke. In some people, smoking dramtically weakens the esophageal valve.

● Try avoiding foods that may be causing your heartburn—fatty foods, chocolate, alcohol, peppermint, onions, cabbage, citrus fruits, chili, coffee and tomatoes.

● Use blocks to raise the head of your bed eight or more inches.

● Use nonprescription antacids.

If these self-care measures don't relieve your symptoms within a week, get help, Dr. McCarthy says. Stomach acid can erode the esophagus, causing painful ulcers. A doctor can prescribe antacids or Gaviscon, a drug that thickens stomach contents so they're less likely to move upward into the esophagus, or drugs to tighten the lower esophageal valve.

Peptic Ulcers

The major symptom of an ulcer in the stomach is a burning, gnawing pain, usually felt throughout the upper part of the abdomen and sometimes in the lower chest. It usually occurs just after eating. The pain can last from half an hour to three hours and can come and go, with weeks of intermittent pain alternating with short pain-free periods.

The more common form of peptic ulcer, the duodenal ulcer, is found in the first part of the small intestine just below the stomach. It produces a similar gnawing pain, usually confined to a small area in the upper middle abdomen, but sometimes radiating throughout. The pain is often temporarily relieved by eating but then returns one to two hours later and lasts for a couple of hours. It's often worst at night. Awakening with abdominal pain around 1:00 to 3:00 A.M. is a strong indication of a duodenal ulcer, although it can also be a sign of other problems, Dr. McCarthy says. What can you do if you're ulcer prone?

● Don't smoke. There is sound evidence that cigarette smokers develop both stomach and duodenal ulcers twice as often as nonsmokers. And because their ulcers heal more slowly and are more likely to recur, smokers more often suffer hemorrhage, perforation and obstruction. "Most of the people coming in for surgery these days are smokers who won't quit," Dr. McCarthy says.

● Avoid aspirin if you have an ulcer. If you must take aspirin, wash it down with plenty of water. In some cases you may need to take an antiulcer medication prescribed by your doctor, Dr. McCarthy says.

● Forget the bland diet of milk, mashed potatoes and custards. It doesn't work. But do avoid whatever foods or beverages make you feel worse.

● Avoid waking up with ulcer pain by forgoing late-night snacks. Instead, take a dose of your medicine at bedtime.

Gallstones

The gallbladder is a pear-shaped sac tucked into the lobes of the liver. It collects bile, a cholesterol-rich digestive fluid secreted by the liver, and pumps it into the small intestine each time you eat.

In many people, bile becomes so saturated with cholesterol that the cholesterol can no longer remain in solution. It forms particles that slowly develop into large stones, says Roger Soloway, M.D., a professor of medicine at the University of Pennsylvania and a gastroenterologist at the Hospital of the University of Pennsylvania. While many people with gallstones have no symptoms, in some people the stones flow out with the bile and get stuck in the bile duct.

The result is a sudden, intense pain in the upper right side of the abdomen that builds to a peak over a few hours, then fades as the stone is either passed or falls back into the gallbladder.

Most likely to get gallstones are women who have been pregnant, overweight people who eat excessive amounts of animal fats, and people over age 60. Young American Indian women are particularly prone, indicating a genetic link. Up to 75 percent of them may develop gallstones.

To decrease the risk of recurrent pain in patients who have gallstones, Dr. Soloway says, doctors have traditionally prescribed a low-cholesterol, low-fat diet. And that still seems to be common advice, although Georgetown University researchers recently found that gallstone sufferers were just as likely to have an attack after a low-fat meal as after a high-fat meal.

Some researchers have associated a high-sugar or refined-carbohydrate diet with increased risk. One study found a high-fiber diet helped by reducing the cholesterol content of bile.

Maintaining the flow of bile through the gallbladder also helps, Dr. Soloway says. Frequent small meals will do this.

People with occasional symptoms do not seem to have other complications of gallbladder disease with any greater frequency than those with no symptoms, research indicates. So today many doctors do not operate unless there is good reason—like recurring pain.

Pancreatitis

The pancreas is a spongy, tapering gland that lies just behind the lower part of the stomach. It makes insulin and important digestive juices.

Pancreatitis occurs when cells in the organ rupture, letting enzymes seep into surrounding tissues, Dr. Soloway says. An acute attack causes agonizing pain in the middle of your stomach. Chronic pancreatitis produces a dull, cramping pain that is aggravated by food and relieved by sitting up and leaning forward. Diabetes and indigestion may also accompany this condition.

Nine times more men than women develop pancreatitis, usually between the ages of 35 and 55. It's almost always associated with heavy drinking or gallbladder disease.

"Giving up alcohol is crucial to the control of this disorder," Dr. Soloway says. Cigarette smoking is also strongly associated with pancreatitis, especially in men. Some doctors call for a low-fat diet. And some prescribe supplemental pancreas enzymes, which reduce the organ's activity and relieve pain.

Irritable Bowel Syndrome

It is estimated that at least half of all patients with abdominal disorders are found to have irritable bowel syndrome (IBS). They have cramps and alternating diarrhea and constipation, but there is nothing physically wrong with their intestines. Symptoms usually appear by age 25, are twice as common in women as in men, and may occur off and on for years, says Nathaniel Cohen, M.D., a New York City gastroenterologist.

Since some other serious digestive diseases have similar symptoms, says Dr. Cohen, your doctor will want to make sure you have none of them. He may do blood and stool tests, and possibly examine the lining of your colon.

Most doctors prescribe bowel-relaxing drugs, bulk laxatives and antidiarrheal medicines for IBS. And an increasing number are taking a look at diet and stress.

Some doctors find their patients get relief by cutting down on sugar, especially in soda, pastries and candy. Barbara Solomon, M.D., a Baltimore, Maryland, internist, finds that 85 percent of her IBS patients respond when they eliminate "food triggers"—which often include milk, wheat, corn, sugar, spicy foods, coffee, tea and alcohol. Many doctors now recommend increased fiber intake to relieve the symptom of constipation.

Some people find their IBS stems from stress. Intestinal muscles actually tighten up and contract into spasm when people are emotionally upset. "People can usually sense when their bowel problems are correlated with stress," Dr. Solomon says. Relaxation training, exercise and biofeedback techniques may all help to modify responses to stress and so reduce IBS symptoms.

Crohn's Disease

Crohn's disease is a chronic inflammation of the digestive tract. Most often affected is the final section of the small intestine, where it joins the large bowel. Periodic cramps and pain in the lower right abdomen (especially right after eating), diarrhea and sometimes a slight fever give this disease symptoms very similar to those of chronic inflamed appendix.

Sometimes the patches of inflammation grow and spread, hindering food absorption. Sometimes they heal but leave scar tissue that can narrow the bowel. Although the disease is uncommon, its occurrence has doubled in the last 20 years. It most often first appears in the late teens or early twenties.

Most doctors rely on anti-inflammatory drugs, painkillers and antidiarrheal medicines to control Crohn's disease. Some, though, see an association with food sensitivities.

"I find that food restrictions work in some cases with inflammatory bowel diseases like Crohn's," Dr. Solomon says. "You limit a few foods and many of the symptoms may be less severe. People find they require fewer painkillers to control their symptoms." Food restrictions won't necessarily cure the condition, Dr. Solomon says, but they can improve it dramatically.

Diverticulosis

Probably one of the most commonly found intestinal abnormalities is diverticulosis, a condition in which the weakened wall of the lower colon bulges outward into tiny, grapelike pouches. Studies have shown that more than half of those over age 60 have diverticulosis. Most never know it, unless their colon is x-rayed for some other reason. But 10 to 15 percent develop inflammation, a condition that is known as diverticulitis, with cramping, bloating, nausea and mild to severe pain in the lower left abdomen.

Diverticulitis can be a serious matter. Most doctors treat it with antibiotics, bed rest and, initially, a low-fiber diet or clear liquids.

But most believe diverticulosis is the result of a low-fiber diet, where the bowel strains to expel small, hard feces. They say the best way to avoid the problem in the first place is with a high-fiber diet, plenty of liquids and prompt heeding of nature's call.

To sum up, what do digestive disease specialists think are the five best things you can do for your tummy? Each has his own favorites, and the list reads like a prescription for overall good health: Eat a high-fiber diet, don't smoke, drink alcohol only in moderation, eat slowly and chew your food well, and investigate any changes in bowel habits.

Angina Relief in a Nutshell

See if you can tell what the people in the following situations have in common.

● Harry has just finished scraping the ice off his windshield. The bitter wind leaves him gasping for air, while a dull ache spreads through his chest, neck and left arm. "Am I that out of shape?" Harry asks himself.

● Emma has been sleeping peacefully for hours. Suddenly she is jolted awake by a squeezing pain in her chest. She suspects indigestion, since playing tennis and jogging have never given her a single ache.

● Jack's dinner of steak and baked potato — with lots of sour cream and butter, of course — was just delicious. So were the apple pie and ice cream he had for dessert. As he pushes himself back from the table, he feels a burning sensation rise up in his chest. "Heartburn," he guesses.

He could be guessing wrong. And so could the others. What these people share are the typical symptoms of angina, a condition so common that it afflicts millions of Americans right now and is knocking on the door of countless others.

"The incidence of angina rises in men from about 4 per 1,000 at age 35 to 44, to 20 per 1,000 by age 55 to 64," says William B. Kannel, M.D., director of the famed Framingham Heart Study and a preventive cardiologist at Boston University School of Medicine. "In women, the incidence starts out lower (1 per 1,000), but they catch up eventually to the men."

If you let it, angina can literally scare you to death. Better instead if it scares you to health. Look at it this way. Angina is a warning sign that your coronary arteries have become narrowed or partially blocked. This narrowing is usually caused by atherosclerosis, the buildup of fatty plaque inside the coronary arteries — the blood vessels that feed oxygen to the heart muscle itself.

Of course, atherosclerosis doesn't occur overnight. It takes a lifetime of bad habits to clog up your arteries, points out Norman M. Kaplan, M.D., author of *Prevent Your Heart Attack* (Pinnacle Books, 1984). Unfortunately, by the time you feel the symptoms of angina, those arteries have narrowed by about 60 percent or more.

Even so, says Dr. Kaplan, symptoms usually occur only when the heart is called upon to increase its work—during physical exertion, after an emotional upset or following a heavy meal. At that time, the heart muscle requires more blood and oxygen than those narrowed arteries can deliver. The result is angina pain—often called exertional angina by heart doctors.

A Signal to Stop

The discomfort or pain is telling you to stop and rest until your heart muscle slows down and regains its necessary supply of blood and oxygen.

It's also telling you it's time for a lifestyle change—time to undo or at least stop the progression of the fatty buildup. That's because if the atherosclerosis process continues and the arteries narrow even further, the flow of blood may be inadequate even when you are at rest. Now that's getting into really dangerous territory.

In fact, the difference between angina and a full-blown heart attack is merely a matter of degree. An anginal episode doesn't leave permanent damage because the lack of adequate oxygen to the heart is only temporary. The pain disappears after a few minutes with rest or drug therapy.

A heart attack, on the other hand, occurs when the oxygen to the heart muscle is inadequate for longer periods of time. Rest or drugs will not automatically make the pain subside and your heart muscle will be permanently damaged, if you should be lucky enough to survive.

Although the exertional type is the most common form of angina, it doesn't explain people like Emma, who have severe attacks during the night while they're asleep, not when they are physically active.

For years there was no clear explanation. Now doctors

have recognized that some people suffer from a condition called coronary spasm, a temporary and involuntary squeezing shut of an artery. Naturally, with blood supply clamped off, the heart screams in protest with angina pain.

"Coronary spasm can occur in people whose arteries are completely free of atherosclerosis, but it's also been found to be associated with the exertional form of angina as well," Dr. Kannel points out. "When patients have pain during exercise and at rest, too, it's often spasm that's causing the resting angina."

Doctors used to think spasm was a rare occurrence—about 2 percent of all angina cases. But now, according to Albert A. Kattus, M.D., of the cardiology division at St. John's Hospital in Santa Monica, California, the estimate of its incidence is around 20 percent.

Serious but Preventable

There's no denying that angina is a most serious condition—life-threatening, in fact. But it lets you know where you stand. You know you have a symptom of coronary artery disease. You know you have a greater chance of suffering a heart attack, a stroke or, worse, sudden death.

Still, there's something even more important that you need to know right now. There are ways to slow your disease—some say even reverse it. Dr. Kannel told us that 40 percent of all angina disappears by itself. "It could be that the people learn to live within their own exercise tolerance. Or sometimes a collateral circulation develops, where smaller arteries take over for the blocked ones, kind of like a self-made bypass," he says.

Yet even if you're in that lucky 40 percent, you should know the latest research concerning your condition. Whether your angina is exertional or spasm, chronic (with predictable episodes of pain) or unstable (where the pain occurs at random or with increasing frequency), there is help. We'll start with diet and end with surgery and cover lots more in between.

The Diet Connection ● The importance of this factor can't be ignored, not with the evidence that keeps surfacing. In one recent study from Denmark, researchers tested eight patients with stable exertional angina by placing them on a low-fat, low (1,400)-calorie diet (10 percent of calories from fat, 15 percent from protein, 75 percent from carbohydrates—mostly complex). Before the experiment began, the patients had been eating a typical high-fat, high (2,000)-calorie Danish diet, say the researchers.

At the end of the three-month study, the patients' cholesterol had dropped an average of 28 percent and their weight was down by an average of 17 pounds. Best of all, exercise testing showed that all the men could stand much more exertion before any chest pain developed than they could before they changed their eating habits (*Lancet,* July 14, 1984).

In another study, researchers from the Netherlands made the dramatic discovery that eating a diet very low in cholesterol (no more than 100 milligrams per day) may actually *reverse* fatty plaque buildup in coronary arteries.

In reporting his findings to the American College of Cardiologists, A. C. Arntzenius, M.D., of the University of Leiden, explained that in about half the patients tested, atherosclerosis had either lessened or at least not gotten worse.

The others in the study did have disease progression, but they also had significantly higher blood cholesterol levels than the patients whose disease was halted.

While you're cutting back on fats and cholesterol, don't eliminate one that's potentially good for you—EPA (eicosapentanoic acid), a factor found in fish oil.

According to a study from Sheffield, England, heart patients who took 10 milliliters of supplemental EPA twice daily for a period of up to two years showed a marked and rapid reduction of triglycerides (a type of blood fat), a decrease in total cholesterol, and an increase in HDL (high-density lipoprotein) cholesterol (the good kind).

What's more, the use of nitroglycerin (a drug commonly used to relieve angina pain) dropped drastically and patients reported fewer episodes of pain, plus an increased exercise tolerance (*Atherosclerosis,* vol. 50, 1984).

Before we leave the diet topic, we want to say a word about salt. Dr. Kannel says it's possible for a high-salt meal to bring on an angina attack. "Salt makes you retain water and sometimes swell with edema," he told us. "Some people think that the vessel walls themselves swell. This could bring on angina pain, especially if your vessels are near the critical point of closure. Salt retention is also believed to be related to increased blood pressure, which can increase the heart's work load."

Exercise ● Physical activity is important, but there are some very severe restrictions. "Exercise can be deleterious if the diseased heart cannot tolerate the increased stress," says Ezra A. Amsterdam, M.D., author of *Take Care of Your Heart* (Facts on File, 1984). That's why angina patients must start with a modest program that is performed in groups supervised on site by medical or paramedical personnel. But the benefits are worth the effort.

"In patients with coronary artery disease and resultant angina pectoris, the symptom of chest pain typically occurs with effort that raises cardiac activity," explains Dr. Amsterdam, who is director of the coronary care unit at the University of California at Davis School of Medicine.

"Since exercise training produces a lower heart rate and blood pressure for a given level of. . .activity, angina can be averted in many instances by this form of therapy. It may even allow a reduction in dosage of antianginal medication.

"For example, if a patient's heart rate rises to 130 beats per minute on climbing a flight of stairs, and angina occurs, this abnormality can be eliminated by an exercise program which reduces the rise in heart rate. . .to only 115 beats per minute while climbing the same flight of stairs."

Stress Reduction ● "Excessive stress can trigger an angina attack," says James L. Levenson, M.D., assistant professor of psychiatry at the Medical College of Virginia in Richmond. "In some forms of stress the adrenal glands secrete epinephrine— the hormone associated with the 'fight or flight' response. This in turn increases heart rate and blood pressure and hence the work load on the heart. Also, some patients may be more vulnerable to artery spasms at these times," Dr. Levenson warns. "Any of these occurrences has the potential of closing down the arteries, bringing on angina pain."

For those who feel their lives are too stressful, Dr. Amsterdam offers these tips.

● Set aside 15 minutes every day to enjoy by yourself. Do nothing, just relax.

● Work around the stresses you can identify. For example, says Dr. Amsterdam, if you hate phone calls during dinner, take the phone off the hook at that time.

● Assign yourself a whole evening each week where you read, go to a movie, watch TV or do anything else you desire. And don't let anyone keep you from your pleasure.

● If you work, set aside several lunch hours a week for yourself with no business or errands conducted then. Visit the library or a museum or just stroll.

● Remember, if these steps don't reduce your stress, there are many specialized programs to help you cope. Seek them out with your doctor's help.

No Smoking ● If you haven't quit already, be sure to do it now. Sure, you've heard it before, but do you know *why* doctors tell you to kick the habit? It's because tobacco plays havoc with diseased arteries. It's even got a name—tobacco angina.

Researchers have found that cigarette smoking not only seems to accelerate fatty buildup in the arteries, but even one cigarette may cause platelets in the bloodstream to clump together. Worst of all, smoking increases coronary spasm and works against antispasm medicines, diminishing the effects of drug treatment.

"Those with angina who quit smoking have half the death rate of those who continue," adds Dr. Kannel. "And that benefit accrues immediately. It's even better than bypass surgery for cutting death rate."

Belief That You Will Lick Your Problem ● This kind of belief, even to the point of denying that the condition is terribly serious, can actually work in your favor, according to Dr. Levenson. At least it did in a group of patients with unstable angina. "We divided these patients into two groups—deniers and nondeniers—based on their score on a specialized set of questions," Dr. Levenson explained to us.

Despite similar treatment regimens, it took the non-deniers about twice as long to become medically stabilized— pain free for 36 hours (*Psychosomatic Medicine,* January/ February, 1984).

Are you a denier or a nondenier? "It's not hard to tell," says Dr. Levenson. "Deniers are people who are less flustered and less frightened by the news of their illness. They'll be lying there in the intensive care unit, smiling. Ideally, they are able to follow all the recommended advice, but still deny the danger they're in. In other words, they're not incapacitated by fear.

"Deniers are people who may flirt with danger; you know, the daredevil types. On a more positive note, they also have a more carefree, jovial attitude toward life.

"Of course, denial can be taken too far, and we watch out for that," says Dr. Levenson. "Continuing to smoke, for example, is downright reckless. On the other hand, when a patient is scared to death, we try to play down their illness a bit, to help them deny it.

"There used to be a tendency by some doctors to try to break through the denial, to make patients own up to their illness. But that is unwarranted when the patient is acutely ill. If denial is protective for the patient, then it's a bad idea to intervene."

Magnesium ● This mineral may be an important factor in preventing spasm angina, say researchers from Israel. They suspect that some spasms might actually be a consequence of low magnesium levels in the blood and tissues around the coronary vessels.

The researchers studied 15 patients over a period of one year. During that time 41 spontaneous episodes of angina occurred. At each attack the doctors injected a solution of magnesium sulfate into a vein. Prompt termination of the attacks was observed within 30 seconds to 2 minutes following each injection. Ordinarily an attack of this type would last 5 to 15 minutes.

Four patients in particular experienced a daily attack for four successive days while in the hospital. Each time they responded promptly to the magnesium sulfate, the doctors report. But after the fourth attack the doctors decided to give the patients additional injections of magnesium sulfate into the muscle every four hours for the next four days. No additional attacks occurred during the next week and the patients were all sent home (*Magnesium,* January/February, 1984).

Medication ● Drugs help prevent attacks of pain, but they are not without side effects. *Nitroglycerin*, the oldest treatment, is placed under the tongue. In a minute or two it dilates the arteries and veins of the body, making it easier for the blood to flow through. Possible side effects include headache, flushing and low blood pressure.

Nitroglycerin also comes in a stick-on patch that provides continuous absorption through the skin for a period of about 24 hours.

Beta-blockers act to slow the heart rate and reduce the force of contraction of the heart muscle. Possible side effects are fatigue, lethargy, impotence and depression.

Calcium channel blockers are the newest drugs to come on the market. They're very effective in preventing coronary artery spasm, probably because they prevent muscles from taking up calcium—a necessary requirement for contraction.

They are also useful for exertional angina, since they lower blood pressure and reduce the work load on the heart. Possible side effects include low blood pressure, nausea, headache and constipation.

Aspirin, although it was never intended to be a heart medication, is recommended by many doctors for angina. That's because aspirin helps keep platelets from clumping together and prevents artery-blocking blood clots from forming.

Also, platelets that don't clump (theoretically) don't release thromboxane A2, a potent artery constrictor—making aspirin potentially useful for spasm angina sufferers.

What's more, those with unstable angina may benefit from aspirin, too. In one study of 1,266 men with unstable angina, those taking one aspirin tablet (324 milligrams) per day had a 51 percent lower incidence of heart attack than the group taking a placebo (fake pill) (*New England Journal of Medicine,* August 18, 1983).

Bypass Surgery ● Most doctors consider this a last-resort option—and with good reason. This is major surgery with a long convalescence. What's more, a study from the National Heart, Lung and Blood Institute indicates that the five-year survival rate of mild to moderate angina patients who underwent the surgery is no better than for those who received only medical therapy.

A newer procedure gaining in popularity, says Dr. Amsterdam, is the percutaneous transluminal coronary angioplasty—also called the balloon procedure. Doctors have found that in some angina patients the insertion and inflation of a special balloon catheter into a narrowed artery is enough to relieve the symptoms of angina. It also requires a shorter hospital stay than bypass surgery.

Of course, if you don't do something about the cause of your clogged arteries, you're still only putting off the inevitable.

Where do you stand now? Are you on a collision course with angina? Are you increasing your risks by eating a high-fat, high-cholesterol diet? Do you run yourself into the ground with work and stress? Do you smoke? Get no exercise?

"We can identify potential victims of angina and heart disease," says Dr. Kannel. "We can tell you if you have an accelerated rate of atherosclerosis."

But it's up to you to change your own lifestyle if you want to beat the odds.

Save Your Life with a Tape Measure and a Minute

In the pursuit of health and well-being, you see your dentist twice a year, get periodic medical checkups, eat right and exercise. But do you E.Y.B.S.O.Y.B.? It's a painless procedure. You don't have to leave home and you don't need any costly equipment. All you need is a full-length mirror, a good light, a tape measure or ruler, pen and paper and the cooperation of a family member or friend.

E.Y.B.S.O.Y.B. (examine your birthday suit on your birthday), advises the Skin Cancer Foundation, and you greatly enhance your chances of avoiding the conversion of a mole into a malignant melanoma. Such melanomas are a life-threatening kind of skin cancer and their incidence is increasing more rapidly than any other form of cancer in the United States—except lung cancer in women.

If you have moles on your body—and according to Jean-Claude Bystryn, M.D., professor of dermatology at New York University School of Medicine and director of its Kaplan Cancer Center Melanoma Program, practically all of us do—don't ignore them and don't panic. Just keep tabs on them. Any change in the way they look or feel is a signal to see your dermatologist—pronto!

"Most moles are benign and do not have to be removed, but there is a bad skin cancer that can develop from a mole," Dr. Bystryn cautions. "As many as 10 percent of the type recognized only within the past few years as dysplastic nevi do become cancerous. And when a mole turns to cancer, it's a melanoma, the dangerous kind that can metastasize. The most common skin cancer, basal cell carcinoma, is different. It may spread on the skin, but not to other organs."

But here's the good news! You can minimize the risk of serious complications if you act in time. Nearly 100 percent of *early* melanomas can be cured by surgery alone.

Yet, "it is estimated that 1 out of every 185 Americans will develop a malignant melanoma during their lifetime," Darrell S. Rigel, M.D., instructor of dermatology at N.Y.U. and editor of *The Melanoma Letter,* declares. "As many as 6,000 will die from this disease and 10,000 will have to undergo extensive surgical procedures and resultant deformities."

Dermatologists concur that this is a tragedy of neglect that could easily be avoided.

And that's where E.Y.B.S.O.Y.B. comes in. Here's how the Skin Cancer Foundation suggests you go about it.

Head-to-Toe Inspection

In front of a full-length mirror, study your birthday suit objectively. Learn where birthmarks and moles are located. Ask your spouse, a relative or your very best friend to help you catalog the moles in the hard-to-see areas of your body—on the back, buttocks and scalp and between the toes. (Return the favor on the other's birthday.)

To help you keep a "mole" record so you can more readily note changes, draw a reasonable facsimile of your front view and another of your back view on fairly heavy paper. Now, observe and note the location of each mole on your mock-up. Use a tape measure or ruler with millimeter markings (inches would not provide the degree of accuracy required) to determine size. Draw a line from the spot to the margin of the page and record the size in millimeters. Also note the color (tan, brown, dark brown, gray, black, blue, pink, rose, white, flesh-colored) and the shape (round, oval, irregular, indented).

For a ready-made, easy-to-use mock-up, send a stamped, self-addressed, business-size envelope to the Skin Cancer Foundation, Box 561, New York, NY 10156 and request the "Helpful Henry—Happy Harriet Early Warning System" for melanoma.

Because of the importance of early diagnosis and treatment, if you are in what dermatologists classify as the high-risk group, you should examine your skin at least once a month and see your doctor right away if any moles have changed in color, size, shape, texture or sensitivity, or if you have noticed any pain, itching, discharge or bleeding.

Who is in the high-risk group? You are if you have fair skin and a history of significant sun exposure; if you have had a melanoma in the past; if you have a family history of melanoma; or if you have multiple dysplastic nevi (high-risk moles) on your skin.

What to Look For

High-risk indicators include:

● Moles that are multicolored—generally a mixture of tan, brown, black or reddish pink within a single mole. Low-risk moles are usually either tan or brown.

● Individual moles that look very different from one another. Low-risk moles resemble each other.

● Moles with irregular borders that may fade off into surrounding skin. Low-risk moles have clear-cut borders between the mole and the surrounding skin.

● Moles with diameters larger than 5 millimeters. Low-risk moles are usually less than 5 millimeters in diameter.

● High-risk moles generally occur in large quantity (more than 100) and are usually found on the back, although they may occur below the waist or on the scalp, breasts and buttocks. Low-risk moles occur in lesser numbers (usually 20 to 50) and are scattered over the body, generally on the sun-exposed surfaces of the skin above the waist. The scalp, breasts and buttocks are rarely involved.

You should examine not only yourself but your children— especially newborn infants. Some dermatologists believe congenital moles have a slightly greater tendency to become melanomas.

Sun Takes the Rap

Parents should also guard their children from sunburn. In a recent study conducted by Robert Lew, Ph.D., of the University of Massachusetts Medical Center, and Arthur J. Sober,

M.D., of Massachusetts General Hospital, persons who reported painful sunburns during childhood had triple the risk of developing melanoma. Adolescents should take heed as well. Those who suffered painful sunburns before age 20 more than doubled their risk of developing malignant melanoma (*The Melanoma Letter,* vol. 2, no. 2, 1984).

The precise mechanism by which the sun does its damage is unknown, but it is theorized that the sun depresses the body's immune system to such an extent that overexposure may induce melanomas anywhere on the body, even in areas that are rarely, if ever, exposed to its rays. Also, Dr. Rigel notes, the sun may damage the DNA, disarranging the cells and initiating the cancer process.

Don't rely on your healthy-looking tan to guard you against damage from the sun's rays. "Even with a tan, skin damage continues to occur with subsequent sun exposure," says John Knox, M.D., clinical professor of dermatology at Baylor College of Medicine in Houston (*Sun and Skin News,* vol. 1, no. 2, 1984).

"Avoidance of sunburn," Connecticut dermatologist Alan Dattner, M.D., stresses, "is the most important deterrent to skin cancer. Fair-skinned people who burn while taking quick vacation jaunts to the tropics to get a fast tan are likely candidates for skin cancer and should have their moles closely monitored."

If you must work or play in the sun, use a sunscreen to block out harmful sun rays. The Skin Cancer Foundation recommends the use of products with an SPF (sun protection factor) of 15. This means that while you are wearing the sunscreen, it will take 15 times longer for your skin to become red from the sun than it would without protection. For best results, the sunscreen should be reapplied every two to three hours during long sun exposure or after swimming. Also, use a lip balm that contains a sun-blocking agent.

If you frequently go sailing or skiing, you're at great risk from overexposure to the sun, because water and snow reflect ultraviolet light. Most skiers underestimate the potential danger of overexposure to the rays of the winter sun.

Avoid prolonged exposure from 10:00 A.M. to 2:00 P.M.,

when the sun is strongest. Bear in mind that many of the sun's rays can pass through clouds and be reflected from snow or sand. Thus, sunscreens may be needed even on a cloudy day or in the winter.

Avoiding sun-induced damage does not mean becoming an indoor recluse. The sun can be your friend and an important source of vitamin D, needed for strong bones.

How does one avoid the risks and enjoy the benefits of the sun? Remember that it's not exposure but overexposure you must guard against. You'll get all the vitamin D you need if you get 20 to 30 minutes daily exposure to sunlight, says Madhu Pathak, Ph.D., of Harvard's Photobiology Unit. For purposes of maintaining health, dietary vitamin D is just as beneficial as vitamin D derived from the sun, says Michael Holick, M.D., Ph.D., of the Harvard Medical School vitamin D research laboratory. Alternate sources include milk and other dairy products fortified with vitamin D, vitamin D tablets and cod-liver oil.

Even though most moles are more of a nuisance than a disease, Dr. Dattner cautions that taking sensible preventive measures is comparable to wearing a seat belt. You may never need its protection, but neither would you chance doing without it.

Understanding Your Thyroid

Mrs. Brown couldn't quite put her finger on it, but she seemed to be getting old before her time. At age 65 she wasn't quite sure what to expect, but it seemed like her friends had energy to spare while she was running out of steam. Her skin was dry and itchy, and her face looked puffy. She always felt cold. She wondered if she was getting pernicious anemia, as her mother had. But the results of her last blood test had been normal. When she developed leg cramps, she started to suspect circulation problems. When a friend she hadn't seen for some time told her how different she looked and asked if she'd been sick, she finally made a doctor's appointment, all the time fearing some dreadful disease.

Jody felt worn out, too, but in a different way. And she had plenty of reason to feel bad. She was working in a job she hated, trying to make enough money to single-handedly raise her daughter. Her hands had begun to shake, sometimes badly, and she was perspiring more than usual. Her muscles ached when she climbed the stairs or carried groceries. She felt irritable and jumpy.

One day, as she was talking with her supervisor, her heart began to race. Within seconds she felt extremely light-headed and thought she was going to faint. She asked to be taken to a hospital. "My nerves must be completely shot," she was thinking. But that's not what an alert nurse thought.

Both these women had developed a simple, treatable problem—one that certainly affected their quality of life but was far from life-threatening. They both had thyroid problems. Mrs. Brown had developed an underactive thyroid (*hypo*-thyroidism), while Jody had an overactive thyroid (*hyper*thyroidism). Their varying symptoms are understandable once you know the function of this butterfly-shaped gland that straddles the windpipe.

Sets Metabolic Rate

"The thyroid secretes hormones that control your body's rate of metabolism—the speed at which chemical reactions like energy burning and respiration occur," says Lawrence Wood, M.D., a member of the thyroid unit at Massachusetts General Hospital, Boston, and an author of *Your Thyroid: A Home Reference* (Houghton Mifflin, 1982). This means it has a direct effect on how fast you use up calories.

And the thyroid indirectly influences many other body functions—temperature, heart rate, hormone levels and even how well the liver, kidneys, muscles and nervous system function. In fact, no part of your body is known to escape its influence.

Thyroid problems are much more common than most people, including some doctors, realize, Dr. Wood says. Recent surveys show that about ten million people in the United States have either an overactive or underactive gland. About two million of them don't even know they're sick. And many more women than men develop problems. One out of every 12 to 15 women has inherited a tendency toward thyroid disorders. They are especially likely to develop a sluggish thyroid past middle age.

Thyroid problems tend to run in families, along with certain other diseases and symptoms. Some members of a typical "thyroid" family will find their first gray hairs by age 30. Others may be prone to pernicious anemia, diabetes, arthritis, itchy skin, allergies and, among the men, learning disorders, Dr. Wood says. Both an underactive and an overactive thyroid may be symptoms of the same genetic condition. In fact, it's not uncommon for a woman who's had an overactive thyroid at a younger age to develop an underactive thyroid as she grows older, whether she's been treated for the overactive thyroid or not.

The Slow Thyroid

When your thyroid loses pep, all body functions slow down. In piecing together Mrs. Brown's case, for instance, Dr. Wood noticed her pulse was only 60 beats per minute and her reflexes were delayed. She was constipated. And her thyroid felt slightly swollen and a little firm. Blood tests confirmed an underactive thyroid.

Mrs. Brown's treatment proved to be simple but lifelong. She was told to take thyroid hormone medication and have periodic blood tests to check her dosage. In about two weeks her dry skin, puffy face and energy level improved. Even her mood seemed cheerier. In six weeks she was her old self.

Early Thyroid Failure

Patients like Mrs. Brown have fairly obvious thyroid disorders. That's not always the case. "The thyroid can begin to fail so gradually that mild symptoms can go unnoticed for months or even years," Dr. Wood says. Many of these cases go undiagnosed if the doctor tests the blood for only *thyroid* hormones.

He checks for this early slowdown by measuring the blood level of a chemical called thyroid-stimulating hormone (TSH), which is secreted by the pituitary gland.

But if there are no symptoms, why bother to diagnose — or to treat? Because it makes a big difference in how people *feel*, Dr. Wood says. That was proved in a study done at Massachusetts General Hospital. Patients whose thyroid hormone level was normal but whose TSH levels were high were given either a small amount of thyroid medicine or a harmless placebo. Those getting the medicine said they felt better and had more energy even though they weren't aware of feeling sick or tired before they'd started the medicine.

"The problem is that many symptoms of an underactive thyroid can be attributed to aging," Dr. Wood says. "In fact, those symptoms may really reflect a gradual decline in your metabolism due to a thyroid malfunction."

An overactive thyroid develops most often in women between the ages of 20 and 40. Long-term stress may trigger the condition, Dr. Wood says.

Too much thyroid hormone can raise the body's metabolism uncomfortably, making you jittery, weak and intolerant of heat. Its symptoms sometimes include bulging eyes and an enlarged thyroid, called a goiter.

An overactive thyroid can be treated with drugs that prevent the gland from manufacturing hormones. These drugs, however, can have a major drawback: They can lower your resistance to infection. In most cases, your doctor will stop the drug after about a year of treatment. In about one-third of cases, the thyroid will have resumed normal function.

If antithyroid drugs fail to control your hyperthyroidism, your doctor may recommend treatment with radioactive iodine, Dr. Wood says. The iodine concentrates in the thyroid, destroying some of its cells. Extensive monitoring of this treatment for more than 40 years has found no increased risk of cancer, either for the thyroid or for any other part of your body. The major problem with radioactive iodine, Dr. Wood says, is that people treated this way often end up later with an underactive thyroid.

Surgery is usually reserved for those who won't or shouldn't take radioactive iodine. It's tricky surgery that can damage the nerves to the vocal cords unless it's performed by a skilled surgeon, Dr. Wood warns. "I'd opt for radioiodine unless I was sure the surgery would be done by an expert," he says.

What about Iodine?

Thyroid problems can sometimes be caused by excess iodine. The thyroid needs iodine to make its hormones, but thanks to iodine in salt as well as many other foods, iodine-deficiency goiter is nonexistent in the United States today, Dr. Wood says. If anything, the problem is too much iodine. The salt-laden American diet contains eight times the Recommended Dietary Allowance (RDA) for iodine of 150 micrograms daily.

Dr. Wood says thyroid problems can develop in sensitive people who take kelp tablets or iodine-containing medicines or are exposed to iodine-based x-ray dyes. Symptoms can appear two to three weeks after exposure. If you know you have a thyroid problem, remind your doctor to limit your exposure or to be on the lookout for symptoms, Dr. Wood suggests.

Sex and the Problem Thyroid

Doctors have known for some time that severe thyroid disorders cause menstrual problems. Now they're beginning to see that minimal thyroid problems can also cause menstrual irregularities. In fact, menstrual problems can be the first, and sometimes only, symptoms of a thyroid problem, says Sheldon S. Stoffer, M.D., a Southfield, Michigan, endocrinologist with a special interest in thyroid and sexual function.

An underactive thyroid can cause heavy menstruation. "I've seen this condition really improve in women placed on thyroid medication," Dr. Stoffer says. Hyperthyroidism generally causes lighter periods and lengthens intervals between periods. It can also cause missed periods and symptoms that mimic menopause.

Hypothyroidism, and its often-accompanying depression, can blunt sexual desire in both men and women, Dr. Stoffer says. In men, hyperthyroidism could be a problem because estrogen levels are elevated. Some men with this condition develop enlarged breasts, which shrink with treatment.

Women with hyperthyroidism, or those taking thyroid medication in dosages that are too high, can have fertility problems, Dr. Stoffer says. He recently saw two women who had been under the care of fertility experts for months. Both promptly became pregnant when their thyroid dosage was reduced.

Today sensitive, effective tests of thyroid function are available. If you have menstrual or fertility problems, especially if you have a family history of thyroid disease, it would be wise to have your thyroid function tested.

Fat? Don't Blame Your Thyroid

It's true that someone with an overactive thyroid can lose weight even when eating normally. The metabolism is so revved up that the body burns calories very quickly. And it's also true that an underactive thyroid can cause people to gain a few pounds, mostly from fluid retention.

But any big weight gain in people with hypothyroidism comes from too much eating and too little exercise, Dr. Wood says. "The proof is that people who are put on thyroid medication don't automatically begin to lose weight. They may lose a few pounds of water, but they aren't going to suddenly start burning off their fat." The good news is that once these people are started on supplemental thyroid, they often feel so much better physically and mentally that they're motivated to go on a diet, and they have enough energy to start an exercise program.

What about Thyroid Cancer?

Thyroid cancer is rare, but in recent years there has been a flurry of thyroid cancers in people who had radiation therapy of the head or neck decades earlier for conditions like enlarged tonsils or thymus gland, or for acne. About one to two million people had such treatments between 1920 and 1960.

To find out if you've had such treatment, write to the hospital where it may have occurred. If you have had such treatment, it's important to get a careful examination, followed by yearly checkups, Dr. Wood says. Your risks don't decrease with time. Your checkup should include a test for hypothyroidism. Most thyroid cancers are successfully treated with some combination of surgery, medicine and radioactive iodine.

Mastering Migraine

"I awake with a small, vague ache behind one eye—the prelude to agony. Then light—any kind of light—hurts me, makes me want to crawl under a rock. I pull down the shades and turn away from the slightest glare.

"Then I see dancing, pulsating starbursts in the air, and the pounding pain behind my eye grows sharper, creeping toward the back of my skull. After that, the least scent of perfume or cigarette smoke makes me vomit. The tiniest noise grates against my nerves. I walk like a drunk, bumping into doorjambs and the corners of tables.

"And worst of all, once the pain begins, nothing can stop it. And when it's going full force, I just want to curl up and die."

This is one migraine sufferer's affidavit of misery—an agony common to a long line of people, from Julius Caesar to Charles Darwin to Virginia Woolf to millions of present-day victims.

This torment can last hours or days, occur every week or twice a year, hurt like a mild toothache or a knife in the brain—it varies from person to person and attack to attack. But *migraineurs* (migraine sufferers) know this for sure: The discomfort called migraine is no ordinary headache.

In fact, migraine is much more than just a pain in the head. In classical migraine (affecting 10 to 20 percent of migraineurs), the actual headache is preceded by a so-called aura of strange nonheadache symptoms. There may be partial blindness, visual distortions (like flashing lights or zigzag patterns in the field of vision), tingling, slurring of words, confusion, sweating, dizziness or bizarre changes in hearing, touch or taste. And when the headache finally comes, it usually (but not always) arrives as a dull ache on one side of the head, growing into a deep, throbbing pain often punctuated by nausea and vomiting.

In common migraine (the type experienced by about 80 percent of migraineurs), there's no warning aura—just the onset of a headache phase like that experienced in the classical mode.

153

Experts say that all this migraine distress is associated with the swelling and narrowing of blood vessels inside and outside the brain. But no one yet knows how or why. Investigators are following up all sorts of leads, but despite all the research on the problem, nobody has found a cure.

There are, however, lots of remedies—some with scientific backing, some without; some highly effective in preventing or aborting migraine attacks, some completely worthless. Here's a rundown of some therapies, both offbeat and conventional, that have helped migraine victims.

Biofeedback

Clinicians report that with biofeedback many migraineurs have had great success in heading off or curtailing migraine attacks, and thus weaning themselves away from migraine medication.

"We've monitored the symptoms of hundreds of our patients with migraine—both before they received biofeedback training and after," says Jack C. Hartje, Ph.D., director of the Hartje Stress Clinic in Jacksonville, Florida. "Using what they had learned to forestall attacks, patients with common migraine averaged a 75 to 80 percent reduction in pain. And classical migraine sufferers averaged an 85 to 90 percent reduction."

Through biofeedback, migraineurs learn to raise the temperature of their fingers or hands simply by thinking about it, thus increasing the blood flow to them. The theory is that this change in blood flow draws blood from the head, shrinking blood vessels there and so reducing migraine symptoms.

Dietary Changes

Some migraineurs are convinced that certain foods can trigger a migraine attack, and scientific research is beginning to back them up. Consequently, major headache clinics routinely advise their migraine patients to drop trigger foods from their diet.

"Many migraine sufferers seem to have an intolerance for foods that are vasoactive—foods that can influence the diameter of blood vessels, especially in the head," says R. Michael Gallagher, D.O., director of the Medical Center for Headache in Moorestown, New Jersey. "Among these are alcohol, caffeine products, cheese, beans, citrus fruits, nuts, pickled foods, nitrite-containing foods, chocolate, grapes, onions and foods containing monosodium glutamate (MSG)."

Other experts—and many migraineurs—accuse these same foods of instigating migraine attacks. So should you automatically exclude all these dietary defendants from your life? No, says Marcia Wilkinson, medical director of the City of London Migraine Clinic and author of *Migraines and Headaches* (Arco Publishing, 1982).

"To find out whether a particular food triggers an attack," she says, "the best thing for you to do is to exclude one food only from your diet for a period of one month and then see whether your headaches are significantly better. This can then be repeated with each of the other foods and drinks."

Sleep Modification

For some migraine sufferers, sleep can be both blessing and curse. Blessing: If you can manage to fall asleep at the onset of an attack, you may awaken pain free. Curse: If you sleep too long (on the weekends, for example), you may instigate an attack. Or even too little sleep (as when you burn the midnight oil) may bring on the pain.

Headache doctors say that oversleeping can trigger migraine attacks in at least two ways—by allowing too much carbon dioxide (a blood vessel dilator) to accumulate in the blood or by forcing changes in the body's level of blood sugar. And fatigue brought on by lack of sleep is a known migraine trigger.

The prescription for these ills is obvious but often hard to swallow: Maintain regular sleep patterns throughout the entire week, getting no more and no less sleep than your body demands.

Magnesium

Researcher Kenneth Weaver, M.D., of the Quillen-Dishner School of Medicine at East Tennessee State University, says that magnesium therapy may be a potent antidote for migraines, especially in women. He selected 500 women suffering from migraines (300 of whom were pregnant) and asked them to take 100 to 200 milligrams of magnesuim each day. He found that 70 percent of them soon stopped having migraine attacks, and another 10 percent showed improvement in migraine symptoms.

"These patients got relief very quickly, in a matter of a few days or even hours," Dr. Weaver claims. "Some of the women reported that they had had migraine headaches for two weeks straight, but became symptom free after taking magnesium supplements. These results, of course, have to be confirmed by further research."

Hot/Cold Therapy

Since the diameter of your blood vessels can be altered by exposing them to heat and cold, can you use heat and cold to reduce migraine symptoms? There's no scientific evidence that you can, and most headache experts are skeptical. But a few migraineurs claim that they've been able to abort a migraine attack with this kind of therapy.

Augustus S. Rose, M.D., professor emeritus of neurology of UCLA School of Medicine, advocates hot-and-cold showers and says that for some patients they work well. He suggests that at the onset of an attack, you take a long, hot shower, followed by a cold shower that leaves you shivering (though the experience is guaranteed not to be much fun). Often, he says, this method can actually short-circuit the impending pain.

But hot-and-cold showers aren't for everyone. Elderly people and others with certain diseases should avoid them. For these people, says Dr. Rose, crushed ice in the mouth and throat can sometimes accomplish the same thing as a shower.

Medication

Like many headache experts, Joel R. Saper, M.D., and Kenneth R. Magee, M.D., authors of *Freedom from Headaches* (Simon and Schuster), clearly recognize the two sides of migraine drugs. "Ideally," they say, "it would be safer to treat symptoms without having to resort to taking medications. But most migraine patients require medicine to achieve the maximum relief."

Some medications (like analgesics, sedatives and vasoactive

drugs) are used to abort migraine headaches in progress. Others (like antidepressants and tranquilizers) are supposed to prevent migraine attacks from getting started. If your headaches come once in a while, your doctor may prescribe the first type of medication. But if your headaches come fast and furious, he may give you preventive drugs to avoid the side effects caused by too-frequent use of the abortive agents.

At any rate, you should understand that you may not respond to a migraine drug the same way another migraineur does. And above all, you and your doctor must weigh the benefits of such medication against its possible side effects.

Avoiding the Environmental Factors

Studies suggest, and some migraine victims swear, that there are migraine booby traps all around us—factors in the environment that trigger attacks in certain migraineurs.

These instigators include bright or flickering light (like sunlight, fluorescent lighting, television), intense odors or vapors, high winds, loud noises, traveling and changes in humidity, air temperature, altitude or barometric pressure. Some people have even implicated the hot, dry air of a sauna.

Renowned headache doctor Seymour Diamond, M.D., executive director of the Diamond Headache Clinic in Chicago, says that migraine sufferers can learn to avoid trigger factors by keeping a "headache calendar." It's a record of the date and time of each headache, the food and drug intake the day before, and any activity or factor in the environment that could have provoked it.

Stress Reduction

Many migraine sufferers know all too well that stress can kick off an attack. In *Advice from the Diamond Headache Clinic* (International Universities Press, 1982), Dr. Diamond and a colleague explain, "In times of emotional stress, certain chemicals are released that provoke the vascular changes that cause a migraine headache. The attacks become more frequent in periods of increased stress. Factors related to stress include anxiety, worry, shock, depression, excitement and mental fatigue.

"Repressed emotions can also precipitate migraine headaches, and the muscle tension often brought on by stress situations can add to the severity of the headache. After a stressful period there may be a letdown which can, in itself, trigger a migraine headache. The arteries may be constricted by prolonged stress, and when the individual is finally able to relax, the blood vessels may dilate, causing the headache," they write.

Unfortunately, the preventive for stress-induced attacks goes against the grain of modern life: relaxation and stress control. But these factors are essential parts of antiheadache programs in many major clinics.

"To prevent stress-induced migraines, we try to teach our patients to avoid stressful situations and to control their emotional reactions to them," says Thomas J. McQueen, Ph.D., a behavioral therapist at the Physicians' Headache Clinic in Tampa, Florida. "And part of this training involves relaxation techniques—methods for reducing emotional and physical tension before it has a chance to trigger a migraine."

Cholesterol Clean-Up Time

Human beings can't live without it, yet it may be partly responsible for one out of every two deaths in the United States. An essential body chemical, it is the building block of cell membranes, sex hormones, digestive tract bile acids and vitamin D. Yet, in excess, it can cut off blood supplies to the heart or brain.

It's cholesterol, and what you don't know about it can hurt you.

Though about 20 to 30 percent of the circulating cholesterol in the body comes from animal fat in the diet, the rest is manufactured by the liver. Americans eat about twice as much cholesterol as they need. Though the dietary glut signals the liver to produce less, it's a case of too little, too late. So the excess cholesterol, a white powder encased in buoyant capsules of fat and protein called lipoproteins, is carried through the bloodstream, where it clusters, like so much fish roe, in the walls of arteries.

The surplus cholesterol itself may damage the cells of the endothelium, the delicate inner lining of the artery. But the arteries may have already been left vulnerable by the pounding of high blood pressure or oxygen deprivation caused by cigarette smoking. In the presence of high cholesterol, and possibly as part of a repair process, smooth muscle cells filled with droplets of cholesterol proliferate and lay down a network of connective tissue in the artery wall. This becomes the basis of an arterial buildup called plaque.

In time, this plaque can calcify, hardening like plaster. In fact, English physician Edward Jenner, developer of the smallpox vaccine, once reported that during an autopsy his scalpel struck something hard and gritty. To his horror, he discovered the "bony canal" that notched his knife was an artery.

But long before they turn an artery hard and brittle as coral, these arterial plaques, part of a disease called atherosclerosis, clog a vessel the way fat and food scraps stop up a kitchen drain. Atherosclerosis, a progressive condition that may begin as early as infancy, can cause complications (ranging from heart attacks to strokes) that usually don't appear until middle age. These complications account for one out of every two deaths and are the leading cause of permanent disability in the United States. Yet, in most cases, atherosclerotic disease can be lessened.

Plague of Affluence

Though there may be a strong genetic factor in the development of atherosclerosis, it is in large part a lifestyle disease. It appears to be the plague of affluence, affecting mainly Western industrialized countries where animal-fat diets are the best that money can buy. But the diet connection was long in coming. One of the many clues that led to the confirmation of its role in heart disease was a drop in coronary heart disease deaths in Europe that coincided with World War II rationing. The rate climbed again when Europeans were able to restock their pantries with the once-scarce meat, eggs and butter, leading scientists to examine how dietary fat affected the heart.

For many Americans, their subsequent findings mean that early intervention and treatment can start at the dining table. And it apparently has. In fact, several medical experts believe there is a direct connection between the decline in Americans' consumption of cholesterol and saturated fats and a drop in the death rate from coronary heart disease in the last two decades.

One of those experts is W. Virgil Brown, M.D., of the Mount Sinai School of Medicine in New York. Dr. Brown believes that one-tenth to one-third of the 26 percent decrease in heart attacks over the last 20 years may be diet related. The decline in the death rate, he notes, occurred simultaneously with a reduction in the consumption of cholesterol and saturated fat and a 75 percent increase in the use of polyunsaturated vegetable oils, which reduce serum cholesterol. At the same time, average cholesterol levels declined at least 5 percent.

"Though genetic factors are very important," says Dr. Brown, "I believe that for the great majority of people, lifestyle changes should be enough to eliminate cardiovascular disease."

Daniel Steinberg, M.D., Ph.D., is director of the specialized center of research on arteriosclerosis at the University of California at San Diego. Last year he chaired a diverse panel of experts brought together by the National Institutes of Health (NIH) to arrive at a consensus on what, if anything, could be done about cholesterol. Among their findings after two days of viewing and dissecting the evidence was that most Americans can achieve a 10 to 15 percent reduction in serum cholesterol by diet alone.

The 15 percent figure may appear insignificant, but this is deceptive because large population studies have shown that a 1 percent decline in serum cholesterol may produce a 2 percent decline in heart attacks and sudden death.

"If our extrapolations are valid," says Dr. Steinberg, "that can mean a 20 to 30 percent decrease in the incidence of coronary heart disease. It could save as many as 100,000 lives this year."

The panel endorsed a diet for all Americans based on the

American Heart Association (AHA) diet, which derives no more than 30 percent of its calories from fat. Most people consume a diet that is 40 percent fat. The diet also stipulates no more than 10 percent of a day's calories should come from saturated and 10 percent from polyunsaturated animal and vegetable fats. It also recommends that cholesterol intake be reduced to 250 to 300 milligrams a day, a figure aimed at keeping serum cholesterol at safe levels, considered under 200 milligrams per deciliter, which is how serum cholesterol is measured.

(It is easier to understand those figures once you realize that for every extra 100 milligrams of cholesterol per 1,000 calories you eat, there's an average increase of 3 to 12 milligrams per deciliter of circulating blood cholesterol. That means that if you eat one extra egg—containing about 275 milligrams of cholesterol—on a 1,000-calorie diet, you could have an increase in blood cholesterol of about 8 to 32 milligrams per deciliter. That may not be of any consequence if your cholesterol hovers around 160, but could be important if it's 220 or more.)

Reducing the Risk

Today, more than half of all adult American men have blood concentrations over 200 milligrams per deciliter, meaning they have entered what the American Heart Association calls "the zone of accelerating risk" for heart attack. (Women, in general, tend to have lower serum cholesterol.)

Coronary heart disease is common in countries where blood cholesterol exceeds 200 milligrams per deciliter and exceedingly low in countries where cholesterol concentrations are about 60 percent as high.

The NIH-AHA diet represents a crucial change for the average American man, who would have to eat about half as many eggs as he does now, as well as one-fifth less meat, poultry and fish and one-sixth less fats and oils. Though there has been a significant decline in the consumption of beef and eggs, they still remain the largest single contributors to dietary cholesterol intake, according to U.S. Department of Agriculture (USDA) figures.

Strict though the diet may be, it could save your life if you're among the half of the American population at risk. "Obviously, if you don't die of heart disease you die of something else," says Dr. Steinberg. "But it's nice to have the option."

There is a way to customize a heart-saver plan for yourself, starting with a risk assessment that will require you to have a cholesterol screening. Once you know some specific details about your blood cholesterol, you can better assess your risk of atherosclerosis and its deadly complications.

But cholesterol isn't the only gauge. Your age, sex, family background and habits each play a role. A cholesterol count of 220 milligrams per deciliter may not be as significant, for instance, if you have no family history of cardiovascular disease, aren't overweight, diabetic, hypertensive or sedentary, don't smoke or aren't an older man or postmenopausal woman, all recognized risk factors for coronary heart disease. Though you're wise to adopt the diet anyway—it can only help—you may find you want to direct even more of your energy to losing weight or exercising.

Types of Cholesterol

The first thing you want to do, of course, is get the whole picture. Once you know your total serum cholesterol concentration, you want to know what kinds of cholesterol are most abundant in your blood. It makes a difference.

When a blood sample is spun in a centrifuge, the cholesterol-carrying lipoprotein particles are separated into layers according to their density. One layer is composed of high-density lipoproteins (HDL), combining protein with about 25 percent fat. A second layer is composed of low-density lipoproteins (LDL), proteins that contain about 75 percent fat and are, in fact, large, oily particles considered the major carrier of blood cholesterol. There is another, less studied, cholesterol-containing particle called an intermediate-density lipoprotein (IDL). To further complicate matters, there are two known subfractions of HDL—HDL_2 and HDL_3—and another particle known as a very-low-density lipoprotein (VLDL), which is made up mostly of triglycerides, another blood fat.

What is important to know is that high levels of the large fatty molecules known as LDL are linked to increased risk of heart attack. More than half of the people in Western industrialized nations have LDL levels that put them at high risk. In fact, according to one source, high LDL is so prevalent that it is considered statistically "normal."

On the other hand, HDL, particularly HDL_2, seems to exert a protective effect, possibly by preventing cells from absorbing cholesterol or by actually removing cholesterol from cells and transporting it to the liver, which clears it from the body.

Having a favorable (relatively high) ratio of HDL to total cholesterol, as most premenopausal women do, is considered a good omen. Like a high ratio of HDL to LDL, it means a decreased risk of coronary artery disease. But what is under investigation as an even better heart-disease predictor is the amount of IDL in the blood, says Ronald Krauss, M.D., staff senior scientist at the Donner Laboratory of Medical Physics at the University of California, Berkeley.

IDL is a precursor of LDL, a kind of raw material from which this deadly form of cholesterol is made. But, says Dr. Krauss, it is "biochemically and functionally" different from LDL. "It's a larger particle, contains more cholesterol and could be viewed as more atherogenic," he says.

In fact, Dr. Krauss and his colleagues found that over a two-year period, the change in the level of IDL in the blood of 63 men with elevated cholesterol and evidence of coronary artery disease was as reliable an indicator of coronary artery disease progression as the ratio of HDL to LDL.

"IDL may be a highly specific predictor," says the researcher. "In fact, it may be more directly connected to the process of atherosclerosis than LDL or the HDL:LDL ratio."

Unless your blood fat levels are regulated by some errant gene and require drug therapy, you have tremendous power not only to lower total blood cholesterol and LDL but to increase HDL and potentially reverse the progress of atherosclerotic disease. Diet, exercise, weight control and giving up cigarettes may alter the condition of your arteries. And most experts agree there's a good place to start.

Reduce Saturated Fats ● Excessive amounts of saturated fat in the diet tend to increase the level of blood cholesterol even more than cholesterol-rich foods such as eggs and organ meats, which should also be restricted. The cholesterol contents of beef, poultry and some fish are almost identical. What makes poultry and fish so desirable on heart-saver diets is that they are low in saturated fats. "Saturated fat is *the* important component," says Dr. Steinberg. "The changes you effect by changing the saturated fat content of your diet are the important ones."

Saturated fats, with few exceptions, are found in animal products. Studies with animals, including primates, have shown that diets low in saturated and other fats can lead to regression of atherosclerotic plaque. "There is some anecdotal human data, case reports of arterial lesions going away with diet and changing several risk factors simultaneously, such as smoking and weight loss," says Dr. Brown. "There's no large study showing a significant number of lesions regressing over time, but there are some potential studies going on now."

Scientists do know that human beings who lower their intake of saturated fats and substitute polyunsaturated fats like corn or safflower oil, which tend to lower serum cholesterol, do have lower levels of LDL cholesterol with little if any significant change in HDL levels.

If you're the meat-and-potatoes type, trimming saturated fat from your diet may not be entirely painless. "You simply have to choose lean cuts of meat and try not to eat meat more than three times a week," advises Dr. Steinberg. Though there's about the same amount of cholesterol in a lean cut of beef as in an untrimmed one, there are less saturated fat and calories, which are the more important factors to consider.

Poultry and fish, with far fewer calories and saturated fats, are fine beef and pork substitutes. "Most fat is marbled through beef so it's more difficult to control it," says Marjorie Whelan, R.N., coordinator of the center for human nutrition at the University of Texas Health Sciences Center. "With chicken, you can peel off most of the fat with the skin."

With some fish—mackerel and salmon, for instance—the

fat is important. These fish contain certain fatty acids that have been shown to lower serum cholesterol. One study showed that people who ate a salmon-rich diet for four weeks lowered their total blood cholesterol by 15 percent although they were eating 500 milligrams of cholesterol a day.

How you cook meat can also reduce the amount of fat and cholesterol you eat. "Broiling meat in a roasting pan that allows the fat to drip down rather than soaking back into the meat is a wise idea," says Dr. Steinberg.

Butter can be replaced by margarine and low-fat cheeses substituted for those creamy Bries and snappy Cheddars that add fat and calories to the diet. And believe it or not, skim milk can become an acquired taste. "With my own kids, who claimed to hate the taste of skim milk, I spiked their milk, first with 25 percent skim milk, then 50 percent," admits Dr. Steinberg. "In six months, I had them drinking it straight. Now when they have whole milk, they say, 'Oooh, too rich.'"

Exercise ● There is some evidence that exercise can raise levels of HDL cholesterol and lower levels of LDL. And you don't have to run marathons to see an improvement. "All you need is what's described as aerobic exercise," says Ms. Whelan. "Not vigorous, just moderate walking, running or biking three times a week for half an hour."

Researchers at the Washington University School of Medicine found that older men (average age, 60) who exercised regularly had HDL levels that were markedly higher than those of groups similar in age who did not exercise and those of a group of younger men.

Exercise—along with diet—can also help eliminate another serious heart disease risk factor: obesity. However, according to researchers at the Stanford Heart Disease Prevention Program at Stanford University, physical activity has an effect on blood fats independent of its effect on body size (although, at least in runners, the increase in HDL appears to be associated with lower body fat). Interestingly, in the Stanford study, the 14 sedentary men, ages 36 to 54, who took up a running program reaped several benefits in addition to lower total cholesterol and higher HDL. They lost weight while increasing their carbohydrate consumption along the lines suggested by the U.S. Dietary Goals to help reduce heart attack risk.

Stop Smoking ● Cigarette smoking is linked to low levels of HDL cholesterol and oxygen deprivation of body tissues that can damage arterial walls. Nicotine, tars and other chemicals in cigarette smoke also appear to have a deleterious effect on blood vessels and other parts of the cardiovascular system.

Researchers at Oregon Health Sciences University found that smoking could even wipe out the edge women have over men: higher HDL and lower LDL levels. They found that women who smoked had ratios of LDL:HDL and total cholesterol:HDL similar to those of male nonsmokers, a finding not unlike that reported by the well-known Framingham Heart Study. And if you exercise and smoke, you might as well take it easy, because researchers at the University of Louisville discovered that smoking can reduce the HDL-raising effects of an exercise program.

Lose Weight ● An estimated 30 percent of Americans over the age of 40 are overweight. Studies have shown that obese people tend to have low HDL levels. Add to this obesity's link to high blood pressure and diabetes and the higher rate of coronary heart disease in the older age groups and you have a risk factor with a few ugly bonuses.

There is some evidence that weight loss in obese men, though not women, decreases LDL and increases HDL cholesterol. Considering the association between obesity and other serious risk factors, however, weight loss has far more to recommend it than a potential increase in the good cholesterol.

Add Fiber ● Oat bran, corn and beans contain fiber that seems to be particularly effective at lowering blood cholesterol, though precisely how remains a mystery. "You can lower cholesterol 10 to 15 percent over and above any changes you might get by lowering saturated fats," says Dr. Brown. "And you don't need huge quantities—no more than 40 to 60 grams a day of the fiber component itself." What this usually means is doubling or tripling the amount of these foods the average American consumes.

Scientists at the Veterans Administration Medical Center in Lexington, Kentucky, found that oat-bran diets decreased serum cholesterol concentrations by 19 percent and LDL by 23 percent. The men in the study continued the diet at home,

HOW HIGH?

When it comes to cholesterol, how high is too high?

The Pooling Project, the largest study of its kind on blood cholesterol levels, showed that coronary heart disease risk rises sharply over 220 milligrams per deciliter (mg./dl.). The consensus report of a prominent panel of experts convened last year by the National Institutes of Health found that risks begin to climb more rapidly over 200 mg./dl.

Richard A. Carleton, M.D., chief of cardiology at Memorial Hospital and Brown University in Rhode Island, says he would have been "a trifle happier with lower levels." He argues that the incidence of heart disease probably begins to increase at levels over 180 mg./dl. Upper limits are calculated from the mean of what is statistically considered "normal"—and normal for most Americans is already too high, says the physician. "With cholesterol," he says, "it's really bad to be at the U.S. average."

The consensus panel set as its goal a reduction of blood cholesterol to 180 mg./dl. for adults under 30 and about 200 mg./dl. for individuals over 30. And it also established estimated levels of moderate and high risk for most of the population.

Age	Moderate Risk (mg./dl.)	High Risk (mg./dl.)
2-19	greater than 170	greater than 185
20-29	greater than 200	greater than 220
30-39	greater than 220	greater than 240
40+	greater than 240	greater than 260

eating about 1½ ounces of oat bran a day, and continued to have good cholesterol profiles during the two-year follow-up.

Other forms of fiber from fruits, legumes and vegetables are also associated with lower serum cholesterol and, as a bonus, with protection from some forms of cancer.

Try Vitamin C ● Studies have shown that taking vitamin C can result in a decrease in serum cholesterol and may be a particularly effective blocker of seasonal cholesterol increases.

Researchers at a Scottish hospital gave one gram of vitamin C a day to a group of young, healthy volunteers and found that serum cholesterol levels dropped in a matter of two months. An older group given the same dosage had no significant decrease, so the researchers doubled the dose. They saw a similar drop in blood cholesterol at the end of a year, which they attributed not to the large dose but to a longer response time in older subjects.

The same researchers then gave the one-gram dose to a small group of healthy volunteers for a full year and compared them to a similar group who weren't getting any supplemental vitamin C. The volunteers who weren't taking vitamin C had serum cholesterol levels 16 percent higher in January than in June. The vitamin C group had no seasonal fluctuations.

Solving the Mystery of "Referred Pain"

We've seen it in the movies but we forget that it actually occurs: the phenomenon of "phantom pain." A person whose leg or arm has been amputated cries out at the pain or burning he feels in the limb that no longer exists. But the pain, nevertheless, is real—as real as if the limb were still there.

Strange as it may seem, phantom pain is not alone in the medical world. It represents merely one of the more sensational examples of a very common syndrome known as referred pain.

By definition, referred pain is pain that arises in one part of the body but, for no apparent reason, makes itself felt in another part of the body. One result of this ventriloquism of pain is that perfectly healthy tissue may ache while the real problem goes undetected. Not surprisingly, this transference can play havoc with a doctor's attempt to diagnose and treat.

"The place where you are feeling the pain isn't always the culprit," says Gerald M. Aronoff, M.D., director of the Spalding Pain Center in Boston.

"The most common example is the man who is having a heart attack. He grabs his chest, but then the pain radiates down his arm. That's cardiac pain referred to the arm," he says. "It's the same way with neck problems. People may feel pain only in their hands. We have patients who say they need treatment for wrist pain when the real problem is in their neck.

"There are classic cases where a person's nose hurt so badly that he wanted to cut it off, when the real source of the pain wasn't in his nose at all, but in certain nerves of the face. Some people have had all of their teeth removed because of dental pain, only to find out later that the teeth weren't the problem. We have had people with leg pain so severe that they would ask us to cut their leg off, but the real source of the pain was in the muscles or disks of the lower back," Dr. Aronoff says.

Pain specialists have noticed countless other examples of referred pain. "People who have a disease in the area of the hip, such as bursitis, may often report referred pain on the inside of the knee," says Hubert Rosomoff, M.D., of the University of Miami's Comprehensive Pain Center, which has a staff of 80 physicians and ranks as one of the largest pain treatment and research centers in the world. "The pain may occur in the knee and the hip, or it may not be felt in the hip at all.

"People suffering from an intra-abdominal catastrophe, in which there may be a rupture of an organ or an abscess under the diaphragm," he adds, "may complain of pain on the tip of their shoulders."

Referred pain is something that dentists run into all the time, especially dentists who specialize in treating the temporomandibular joint (TMJ), where the jawbone is linked to the temples. Dentists have found that pain created by a misalignment of the TMJ is often referred to other parts of the head or neck.

"The site of the referred pain varies from patient to patient," says Neil R. Gottehrer, D.D.S., a TMJ specialist at Craniofacial Pain Consultants in Philadelphia. "Someone may feel dizzy, or have eye pain, or pain in the neck or shoulder. Each patient is different."

Sometimes TMJ pain appears as far away as the shoulder or arm. "One of my patients had been seeing a neurologist about occasional numbness in his arm," Dr. Gottehrer says. "When he came in here, I touched a point on his cheek and his entire arm immediately went numb. That was proof that the arm problem was referred from the TMJ."

In fact, any shoulder or neck pain that won't go away, Dr. Gottehrer says, might be referred. "If you go to a chiropractor for neck pain and your neck doesn't get better, then you should look at the possibility of referred pain. It's very common."

A knowledge of referred pain comes in especially handy for someone who suffers from low back pain that just won't go away. Research has shown that knots, or spasms, in the muscles of the abdomen, the buttocks and even the legs can refer pain to the lower back. That makes diagnosis difficult. Pain in the soleus muscle, which is near the heel, can also be referred to the lower back. Unless these spasms are detected and massaged away, the lower back pain will persist—even when there is no direct injury to the back (*Postgraduate Medicine,* February, 1983).

The Guilty Shoulder

Shoulder injuries also often go undiagnosed because the pain is referred to the arm. One sports medicine specialist, Ben E. Benjamin, Ph.D., in his book *Listen to Your Pain* (Penguin, 1984), writes that "the tricky thing about evaluating your own shoulder injuries is that it never hurts where it's supposed to."

Dr. Benjamin cites the example of a young gymnast who was unsuccessfully using ice to treat pain in her bicep muscle, just above the elbow. An examination for referred pain showed that the girl had injured a tendon at the top of her shoulder, 12 inches from the site of the pain.

"The five most common shoulder injuries all hurt in about the same place: the middle of the upper arm," Dr. Benjamin says. "The more severe these injuries are, the farther they refer the pain toward the wrist."

Eye pain often turns out to be referred pain, too. The pain is usually referred from the sinuses and typically accompanies a cold or a bout of the flu. A variety of rarer diseases, such as diabetes or cancer, can also refer pain to the eye.

Trigger Points

No one entirely understands how or why the nervous system plays this game with the body, making us guess which shell the real cause of the pain is hiding under. Neurologist Austin J. Sumner, M.D., of the University of Pennsylvania, admits, "We don't have all the answers about referred pain."

But they do have some of the answers. They know about "trigger points." In the course of groping along the skin and probing the muscles of their chronic pain patients, doctors sometimes come across localized tender spots, which they've called trigger points. When they press these spots, their patients feel a stab of pain at the site of the referred pain. Trigger points are often the source of the pain.

Over the years, doctors have discovered that if they inject a local anesthetic such as novocaine into the trigger point, they can relieve the pain temporarily. They've also found that if they stretch and relax the muscle under the trigger point, they can often give the patient relief.

Many of the trigger points are located in tight muscles. Others are located in scars, or in the joints, or in tissues that surround bones. In some cases, lifting heavy boxes or kneeling down to scrub floors or work in the garden for long periods of time can initiate the problem.

Doctors only have a vague idea, however, why the nervous system is so easily fooled into thinking that heart pain is arm pain or that hip pain is knee pain. Dr. Sumner explains that this is probably an honest blunder on the part of the brain. Nerves leading from two parts of the body sometimes converge at almost the same spot on the spinal cord, and the brain can't always tell which of the two places sent the message.

The history of the study of referred pain in the United States involves a physician who worked with President John F. Kennedy.

Janet G. Travell, M.D., who was born in 1901 and still practices medicine in Washington, D.C., worked with cardiac patients in a New York City hospital in the late 1930s and early 1940s. Many of them suffered from severe arm and shoulder pain. By coincidence, she also was suffering from shoulder pain. She had noticed that she could intensify her own pain by pressing an apparently unrelated sore spot near her shoulder blade.

At about the same time, she happened to read two medical articles that described her condition exactly. By poking the shoulder blades of her heart patients, she found that they had the same problem. Following the procedure recommended in one of the articles, she soon found relief and began treating her patients with novocaine and, later, with muscle stretching. At one point she became known as the "trigger queen."

Her work eventually led her in the 1950s to John F. Kennedy, then a senator. It was she who was largely responsible for relieving Kennedy's chronic and often disabling back pain. It is probable that without her help, Kennedy would not have been able to run for president. In 1961, she was appointed White House physician.

What can you do about referred pain if it strikes you? There's a lot you can do.

A wealth of new information about coping with this problem is contained in the book *Myofascial Pain and Dysfunction, the Trigger Point Manual* (Williams and Wilkins, 1983), which Dr. Travell coauthored with David G. Simons, M.D.

This book is written with doctors in mind, and it shows them how to detect and anesthetize trigger points. But it is also full of information that you can use to keep referred pain from returning, as it is wont to do.

For example, higher-than-normal amounts of thiamine (vitamin B_1), vitamins B_6, B_{12} and C and folate are needed to keep pain at bay, Dr. Travell and Dr. Simons say. Likewise, muscles have a special need for calcium, potassium, iron and trace minerals.

Exercise may be even more important. "Exercise to stretch the involved [painful] muscle is the key to relief from myofascial pain," the authors say. Their book illustrates the best ways to stretch out tight muscles and how to do things like open jars and rise from chairs—tasks that can trigger the return of pain.

Finally, help yourself by thinking positively. Anxiety contributes to muscle tension, and depression retards recuperation. An upbeat attitude and a desire to get well can speed healing.

Fitness Newsfront

Walk Your Ills Away

It wasn't very long ago that walking was considered the world's most popular (and only) mass-transit system, but not much more.

In today's world of subways and space shuttles, walking has quite suddenly reemerged — as a mass health-regeneration system.

A regular walking program can help you lose weight, give you more energy and tone your flabby muscles. It can help prevent heart disease, relieve the pain of angina, alleviate mental depression and ease some of the pain of arthritis, as well as reverse some of the physical aspects of aging.

It's hard to believe that something as simple as walking can really produce all these benefits, but scientists are beginning to find that the world's oldest form of aerobic exercise may really be the best. Take its effect on weight loss, for example.

"Regular exercise can be the single most useful thing a moderately obese person can do to lose weight," says Jömel Grinker, Ph.D., professor of nutrition in the School of Public Health and Pediatrics at the University of Michigan. "I tell almost everyone that walking is the best exercise they can get, because it doesn't stress the body the way running does. Swimming is good, too," she adds, "but you need a pool for that."

But why go to all that trouble? Why not just go on a diet to lose weight?

"For one thing, with exercise you don't suffer the decrease in metabolic rate that accompanies severe caloric restriction," says Dr. Grinker, who heads the program in human nutrition at the university. She explains that stringent dieting lowers the body's metabolism, which means that proportionately fewer calories are burned. But exercise helps to *increase* the metabolic rate, meaning that more calories are being burned up over a longer period of time.

There have been many studies showing that exercise is more effective than dieting for losing weight. In one, Grant Gwinup, M.D., assembled a group of obese people in California who had all failed to lose weight by dieting. Dr. Gwinup asked them to continue their normal eating habits but to walk at least 30 minutes or more per day for a year. At the end of a year, all of the subjects had lost weight, averaging 22 pounds each.

One of the big advantages to walking is the *kind* of weight you lose. If you're walking off the bulges, you'll be getting rid of fat, whereas dieting also causes loss of lean body tissue, or muscle.

There is little doubt among health care professionals today that when reasonable eating habits are combined with exercise, such as walking, weight loss is more rapid than when either method is used alone. And with walking you won't get the feelings of weakness and nervousness that usually go along with dieting. While you're walking off unwanted pounds, you'll be doing your heart a favor, too. For many sedentary and older people, brisk walking at a pace of four to five miles per hour can provide a workout for the heart and lungs comparable to that of jogging, according to Robert Kertzer, Ph.D. Dr. Kertzer incorporates walking into a special cardiac rehabilitation program at the University of New Hampshire.

"If the activity is rhythmic, involves a large percentage of the body's musculature and is continuous, it's good for cardiovascular fitness," says Dr. Kertzer, who is an associate professor of physical education at the university.

Joseph Tenenbaum, M.D., a cardiologist and assistant professor of clinical medicine at Columbia University's medical school in Manhattan, concurs.

"The key to therapeutic walking is consistent rhythm in exercise, with major muscle groups kept in action for 30 minutes at least four times a week," he says. "I recommend walking to a lot of my patients."

Many of Dr. Tenenbaum's patients are in the healing phase following a heart attack, and he feels that walking is the ideal exercise for them or anyone who is convalescing to rebuild strength. In fact, Dr. Tenenbaum's patients may be preventing future heart attacks with their walking programs.

Sixty-four patients who had been recommended for coronary bypass surgery by their personal physicians chose instead to try lifestyle modifications. They entered the Pritikin Longevity Center in California for a 26-day session. There, in addition to following the Pritikin high–complex-carbohydrate, high-fiber, low-fat diet, they participated in a walking program of two brisk walks per day, each lasting 30 to 45 minutes.

At the end of the 26 days, all the subjects had lost weight, their blood pressures decreased, their serum cholesterol and triglyceride levels were significantly reduced, and in some cases, angina was relieved. Five years later, those who continued to follow the program's guidelines at home were still benefiting from it. In fact their mortality rate was actually approaching that of the general population.

Good eating habits unquestionably played a role in these patients' progress, but there are many indications that even without dietary modifications, exercise can help prevent heart problems. The American Heart Association, for example, suggests that regular exercise, such as walking, may protect against heart disease.

Even extremely moderate walking, at a pace too slow to provide the cardiovascular benefits of a brisk walk, can raise HDL-C (high-density-lipoprotein cholesterol) levels. Since people with low levels of HDL-C are considered to be especially vulnerable to heart attacks, they'd be well advised to get out for daily strolls. In a recent University of Pittsburgh School of Medicine study, 30 sedentary men exercised at three different levels of intensity for 20 minutes at a time. HDL levels rose just as sharply during low-intensity exercises as they did in high-intensity sessions. But if slow walking is better than no walking, fast walking is the best.

"Just being on your feet and moving from point A to point B is not equivalent to an exercise program," warns Dr. Tenenbaum. "Window shopping, for example, or just moving around at work can't substitute for a brisk daily walk."

The reason most health care professionals recommend setting a vigorous pace during your walking workout is that there seems to be a threshold in the intensity of exercise that must be reached to provide for improvements in the heart and circulation. Fast walking, like any aerobic exercise, will enable your heart to beat fewer times, since it is pumping more blood with each beat.

As if strengthening your heart and keeping you trim weren't enough, walking can promote metabolic changes that may help prevent or manage adult-onset diabetes mellitus by inducing an insulinlike effect on cellular glucose uptake. Furthermore, walking can help to halt bone loss, thereby preventing osteoporosis. And since exercise has been shown to slow degenerative joint changes, walking can prevent or relieve some symptoms of rheumatoid arthritis.

In fact, as far as joints are concerned, walking is frequently the best exercise.

"If a person has a damaged joint or ligament, or the kind of back problem that might be aggravated by jolting, then running may be bad for that person," says Robert Leach, M.D., professor and chairman of orthopedic surgery at Boston University Medical School.

"Even walking produces some impact when the heel strikes the ground, but there is no question that jogging produces more impact force. That won't harm a normal joint, but a disabled joint is better off walking," advises Dr. Leach, who has had plenty of opportunity to study the effect of impact on joints in his capacities as consultant to the Boston Celtics, head physician to the summer Olympic teams in Los Angeles in 1984 and orthopedic surgeon to Olympic gold medal marathoner Joan Benoit Samuelson.

"Walking is a very efficient exercise," Dr. Leach asserts,

"especially in terms of toning muscles and giving people a good feeling."

Help for the Depressed

Psychiatrists, particularly, are beginning to recognize the value of the "good feeling" Dr. Leach refers to. Walking, like jogging, appears to promote increased endorphin production (endorphins are neurohormones that may promote a sense of well-being).

"I recommend brisk walking—rapid enough to condition the heart—for all my patients who are depressed or suffering from low self-esteem," says Ralph Wharton, M.D., a psychiatrist in New York who specializes in the treatment of depression. "Even 20 or 30 minutes a day seems to make a difference. For one thing, going for a walk prevents excessive preoccupation and rumination, and it distracts you from your own inner concerns—after all, you have to look where you're going!"

If one of the things that depresses you is the thought of aging, you've got all the more reason to start walking. In a program involving a group of Canadian men and women in their midsixties who were given endurance training that emphasized vigorous walking, several interesting results were achieved: Body fat was decreased, knee extension capabilities were increased, body potassium levels were increased, and the normal age-related loss of bone calcium was apparently halted. In other words, the best way to reach the fountain of youth is to walk there at a brisk pace.

Try "Health Walking"

"The faster you walk, the better you can feel," says Howard ("Jake") Jacobson, executive director of the Walkers Club of America.

Jacobson's aim is to get us all health walking, an activity that he says is best accomplished by pumping your arms vigorously while you walk. Health walking is a noncompetitive form of race walking, a venerable sport that has been an Olympic event since 1908.

"By moving your arms like a sprinter, you can move faster, which will raise your heart rate higher than normal walking," Jacobson says. "And you'll be using more muscles and burning more calories than joggers, with less risk of injury."

How does the novice start health walking? Jacobson recommends walking rapidly in a normal way but with your arms pumping like a sprinter's. Avoid swaying from side to side, he says, because that slows you down.

Jacobson, a coach to Olympians and author of *Racewalk to Fitness* (Simon and Schuster, 1980), emphasizes that health walking can be done by almost everyone, at any age. Young children in Sweden race walk in school programs. In the United States, 93-year-old Gwen Clark health walks six miles every day in New York's Central Park. If you want to take up health walking yourself, you won't be alone: Approximately 10,000 race walkers and health walkers have joined the Walkers Club of America, an organization that sponsors competitions and free classes across the country.

For information about walking clubs near you or for guidelines on how to start one yourself, write to the Walkers Club of America, 445 East 86th Street, New York, NY 10028. If you enclose $3, they'll also send you "Step Lively," a 16-page illustrated how-to booklet on health walking.

Another good book to help you get your feet moving is *Rockport's Complete Book of Exercise Walking*, written by noted walking authority Gary Yander, who'll help you with walking techniques and designing your own walking program. It's available by sending a check or money order for $8.95 to the Rockport Shoe Company, 72 Howe Street, Marlboro, MA 01752.

To set up your own daily walking program, consult with your doctor first if you have pain or haven't had a checkup in some time. Once you've got the go-ahead, get yourself a pair of comfortable, flexible walking (or running) shoes, preferably with cushioned soles. Start off slowly if you're in poor physical condition, building up to as fast a pace as you can handle. Walk at least 30 minutes a day, three or four days a week. In extremely hot or cold weather, walk in a shopping mall, in the halls of your apartment building or around a track in a gym. Go walking by yourself or with a friend, or get a group together. As well as being good exercise, walking can be just plain fun—and that's the best medicine of all!

If You Must Stand All Day

"I used to stand in one spot for nine to ten hours every day," says Anthony DeFrancesco, a barber from Phillipsburg, New Jersey. "My legs were always tired and sore, and I developed pretty bad varicose veins in one of them. I cut down the number of hours I worked, but that wasn't enough. Eventually there was nothing that could help me but surgery.

"The doctor removed the bad veins along the whole length of my leg, and I missed two or three weeks of work completely. That was 12 years ago. Now the other leg is just as bad, so I've had to cut down to working only three days a week."

Unfortunately, DeFrancesco's story isn't unusual. Many of us, such as cashiers, postal clerks and assembly-line workers, are stuck with staying put all day because our livelihoods depend on it. And unless we take some preventive measures, standing still can move us down the road to a number of persistent health problems.

"Do you know of any animal that stands in one place for hours at a time? It's just not natural," says Steven E. Baff, D.P.M., of New York City. "We're meant to move around."

Unlike walking, standing continuously puts increased pressure on certain muscles and bones. And if you have a foot abnormality (as 80 percent of us do), an upright job can become downright painful. Standing keeps pressure on your feet all day and aggravates existing problems—hammertoes, ingrown nails, bunions, severe calluses and ankle strain. "And the heavier you are," says Dr. Baff, "the more pressure you put on your muscles, bones and circulatory system, and the greater your chances of developing arthritic changes from your hips to your toes."

What's more, according to Rene Cailliet, M.D., director of rehabilitation services at Santa Monica Hospital Medical Center and author of *Understand Your Backache* (F. A. Davis, 1984), the longer you stand, the greater the tendency to pronate your feet, pointing the toes outward and flattening the arches. That can lead to chronic irritation along the inside of your foot, Dr. Baff told us. And hard surfaces, such as concrete, can amplify your problems because they offer no cushion—nothing to absorb some of the shock.

So what can you do if you can't afford to walk off the job? "Change your stance as often as possible," advises Dr. Cailliet. "Get up and down on your toes, and try to keep your feet facing forward. Arch supports might be some help."

"If you must stand on a hard surface, try bringing a square of carpet to stand on," suggests Dr. Baff, "or anything that 'gives' a little." Wearing the proper shoes can help, too, he says. "Running shoes are excellent. So are orthopedic oxfords that lace up. Look for shoes with a wide toe box, good arch support, a strong heel counter and shank, and a rubberized bottom that gives some compression."

"It's a good idea to shop for shoes at the end of the day when your feet are swollen," adds Dennis F. Augustine, D.P.M., director of the Park Avenue Foot Clinic in San Jose, California, and author of *The Foot Care Revolution* (Footnotes Unlimited, 1981). "Buy them ¼ to ½ inch longer than your longest toe, because your feet slide forward when you stand."

If you've tried everything mentioned so far but your feet still throb, there is another option available. Podiatrists have a new diagnostic tool called the electrodynogram, or EDG. Using sensors placed on the feet, the EDG does a computer analysis of how you walk, to identify problems and actually quantify imbalances. Based on the EDG analysis, a doctor can custom-design special shoe inserts called biomechanical orthotics, which are said to neutralize most abnormal forces.

In addition to making your feet hurt, standing makes them *hot*. When your dogs are tired and begin to perspire, they create a warm, moist climate that invites fungus infections such as athlete's foot. The itching, blisters and cracks in the skin can be a constant annoyance, and open sores open the door for more serious infections. As if that's not enough, the really nasty thing about athlete's foot is that once you've had it, it's likely to come back again and again.

"Bathe your feet frequently and powder them to keep them clean and dry," recommends Dr. Augustine. "Bring extra footwear with you so you can change into dry shoes and socks during the day. And rotate the shoes you wear from day to day—they don't always dry out completely overnight."

Out of Circulation

Being stationary can also make you feel like you're literally on your last legs, because it brings your circulation practically to a standstill, the way it did for Anthony DeFrancesco, the barber. It promotes varicose veins and thrombophlebitis—inflamed veins associated with blood clots.

Normally the muscles in your legs squeeze the veins, forcing the blood back up toward your heart. To keep the blood from flowing backward, the veins contain one-way valves. When you don't move, though, there's no massaging action by the muscles, and blood pools in the veins, putting pressure on the valves. The veins lose their natural elasticity and the valves stop functioning properly. The result? Distended veins, swollen, aching legs and feet, cramps, muscle fatigue and even mental fatigue. "Nourishment of the tissues is cut off with the blood supply," says Dr. Augustine. "And less oxygen-rich blood is pumped to your brain. You actually feel less alert."

"Again, try to get up and down on your toes every 15 to 20 minutes for a few seconds," advises Dr. Cailliet. "Working your leg muscles gets the blood moving and takes the load off your veins. If you've got a severe problem, your doctor may recommend an elastic stocking for your entire leg that helps pump the blood back up toward your heart."

"Elevating your feet, especially when you sleep, brings out some of the fluid," says Dr. Baff. "And some people benefit from contrast baths—alternating warm and cold foot baths. Soak your feet for a few minutes in warm water, then a few minutes in cold, then warm again, and so on. It opens and closes the blood vessels, forcing them to work and circulating more blood."

Dr. Augustine recommends a foot bath of ½ cup vinegar in two quarts of water, or an Epsom salt solution to increase blood flow. "Massage and regular exercise also promote circulation," he told us. "Avoid wearing constricting clothing because it cuts off circulation, adding to the problem.

"A hard, nonyielding surface impedes circulation, too. Mats with rubber projections, like doormats, are good to stand on. They not only absorb shock, they also make your feet keep moving back and forth, up and down, as they adjust to the varying terrain. It increases muscle tone and promotes better circulation," Dr. Augustine explains.

Locked into Backache

"When people stand for long periods of time, they tend to lock their knees back, using their joints for support instead of their muscles," says Susan L. Fish, a registered physical therapist, of New York City. "That stresses your joints and can lead to joint damage over time. It also tilts your pelvis forward, throwing you into a swayback posture," she explains. "Your abdominal muscles become stretched in such a way that they can't support you properly. That can make your back ache.

"The first step is to become aware that you're locking your knees back," says Ms. Fish. Then you'll have to learn to keep them "unlocked." It may be uncomfortable at first, because it takes more muscle to hold you up. So you'll need to strengthen your muscles to support you better. The stronger they are, the more apt you are to rely on them.

"Changing postures as you stand is a good habit. But when you shift around, don't stand on one leg at a time," she warns, "because you deprive yourself of the benefit of the other leg. Try to keep the weight evenly distributed.

"I recommend taking 30 seconds each hour to bring your joints through a full range of motion. It takes off the strain. To loosen up, try sitting down, and alternate pulling your knees to your chest one at a time. Raising one foot up on telephone books or a stool is also highly recommended to take the strain off your back," Ms. Fish points out. That tip can help you around the house, too, when you're ironing, for instance, or doing the dishes. You can even open the cabinet under the sink and use it as a footrest.

Poor posture can cause other problems, too. If your head hangs forward and your shoulders are rounded when you stand, that's going to cause neck and shoulder strain. And if you have to lean over a desk, bench or countertop while you work, the problem will be worse.

"Adjust the height of your bench or desk so you don't have to lean over," Dr. Cailliet suggests. "Pull back every 10 to 15 minutes and change positions to take off the strain.

"Standing with your arms held in front of you all day can cause fatigue of the muscles of your shoulder blades. Try to support your arms for part of the day—find a place on which to lean them if you can.

"In general, a good exercise program at home along with postural training can help a lot," Dr. Cailliet says.

Ms. Fish agrees. "A daily exercise program can help you maintain good strength and normal range of motion. Preventing most problems caused by standing is easy, inexpensive and takes only a few minutes each day."

If You Must Sit All Day

Homo erectus earned his place in the anthropology texts by, one bright day in evolution, rising up off all fours. The upright biped was born. Experience tells us it wasn't long afterward that the first chair was invented. After all, even prehistoric man needed to take a load off.

In those days, the average fellow divided his time about equally between gathering food and avoiding being gathered for food himself. These days, however, find the modern biped a desk-bound information processor who supports himself mainly on his derriere rather than his feet. Could this be a new phase of evolution? Could we be witnessing the birth of *homo in cathedra,* man in a chair?

If so, we may as well kiss our bottom half goodbye. As one industrial consultant puts it, every office chair ought to come equipped with a cardboard tag that reads, "Caution: Prolonged Sitting May Be Hazardous to Your Health."

Sitting a health hazard? Though it sounds downright un-American, it's true. Whether you're an armchair adventurer, a confirmed couch potato or simply anchored for eight hours to your desk, you *can* overdose on sitting.

Studies have shown that people who spend a good part of their lives sitting may run a greater risk of developing herniated disks, varicose veins, phlebitis and even colon cancer. Many experts suspect that behind America's astonishing workers' compensation costs ($16 billion, or 1.5 percent of U.S. payroll dollars) are industrial accidents resulting from the cumulative damage of sedentary life. You're more likely to harm yourself by sitting too long in a chair than by falling out of it, they say.

"We've become a deconditioned society," says Joy Randolph, an occupational therapist and vice president of Back Systems, Inc., a Dallas consulting firm that helps companies reduce their workers' compensation costs. "We let ourselves get out of shape and then, one day, we bend and twist to throw a paper in the trash can and feel the sudden onset of back pain. For most of us, though, it's not the act we were performing at the time that caused the back pain. That's only the last in a series of events. When it comes to back pain, it's literally the straw that breaks the camel's back."

This year, for the first time, back pain edged out the common cold as the primary reason for lost work time. And sedentary workers are far from immune to this ailment, which is usually associated with occupations that call for heavy lifting. (In fact, when it comes to days lost from work, people in public administration, who usually lift nothing heavier than a box of paper clips, call in sick more often than farmers, construction workers and craftsmen.)

"Physically demanding occupations do have higher incidences of back problems," says Ms. Randolph. "But when we go into primarily sedentary companies, we still see a high incidence of back pain."

If that challenges your concept of "hard" work, it's because you don't know anything about the physical rigors of sitting. "The assumption has been that people who stand do work and

sitting is rest," says Marvin Dainoff, Ph.D., a psychology professor at Ohio's Miami University, who has done research for
the National Institute for Occupational Safety and Health.
"But actually, sitting can put a lot of strain on the whole body."

The fact is, taking a load off your feet simply shifts the
load elsewhere, usually to your back and your legs. And, for
anatomical reasons, the load is much heavier. When you stand,
the forces pressing on the spine's vertebral disks are relatively
equal. When you bend the spine, as you do when you sit, the
balance is uneven.

You can get an appreciation for the dynamics of sitting by
trying this simple exercise right there in your chair. Move your
whole body away from the backrest of your chair, lift up your
feet and legs so your thighs are slightly raised, and pick up your
arms from the armrest or desk. Your entire body is now being
balanced on two small, bony protuberances in your seat called
the ischial tuberosities. If it feels a little like trying to balance
on the two back legs of your chair, you get the picture. To
maintain any sort of equilibrium when you sit, you've got to
anchor yourself with your feet, legs, back or arms—preferably
more than one of them.

What you probably can't feel—yet—are the back muscles
and spinal column straining under the weight. According to a
Swedish study, sitting with an unsupported back puts 40 percent more pressure on the spinal disks than standing does.
(Walking only adds about 15 percent more.) The weight of
your upper body shifts forward and your back muscles tense to
keep you from toppling over. The spinal disks contain a gelati-
nous nucleus that, under extreme pressure, can be squeezed
out like toothpaste from a tube. A disk in that condition is said
to be herniated. Prolonged sitting can create enough pressure
on the lower back to herniate a disk because it's roughly
equivalent to another sure-fire hernia-causing posture, bending from the waist to pick up a heavy object.

A study done at Yale University found that people who sat
half or more of their time on the job had a 60 to 70 percent
greater risk of herniating a disk than those who were up and
about more often. The risk for people over 35 who had been
sitting on the job for five years or more was 2½ times greater.

Bus drivers, traveling salesmen and heavy equipment operators have more to contend with than prolonged sitting. A study by the same Yale researcher found that people who spend at least half or more of their workday driving are at significantly higher risk of disk injury than those who don't.

"Part of the problem is from sitting, but part of it is from the road vibration," says Ms. Randolph. "Every structure in our body has its own resonant frequency. We've all seen an opera singer hit a high note and shatter a glass. She does it by reaching the resonant frequency of the glass. The same can be applied to a person sitting in a vehicle, particularly heavy earth-moving equipment. The resonant vibration of the equipment—about four to five hertz—is about the same as that of the spine."

Of course, your spine won't shatter like a crystal wine glass, but the vibration and prolonged sitting eventually can degenerate the muscle/disk system that keeps you painlessly upright.

Sitting can also take its toll if you're genetically prone to varicose veins. You can turn a predisposition that responds to preventive care into a condition that requires medical treatment just by too much sitting, says Howard Baron, M.D., a New York vascular surgeon.

"I call it the sitting disease, " says Dr. Baron, author of *Varicose Veins: A Commonsense Approach to Their Management* (William Morrow and Co.).

Sitting virtually stills what's often called the venous or peripheral heart, the muscular system in the legs that pumps the blood back into the heart. If you're sitting, your leg muscles aren't contracting, so your venous blood simply obeys the law of gravity. But when blood pools in the legs, it tends to build up dangerous pressure in congenitally weak veins.

Even if your veins are perfectly strong and healthy, you've no doubt experienced the pins-and-needles feeling in your legs when you've sat too long in one position. It's caused by temporarily sluggish circulation—annoying for the healthy but potentially deadly for a varicose vein sufferer.

The chair you're sitting in may aggravate the problem. "A chair puts unremitting pressure on the backs of the thighs, compressing the veins," says Dr. Baron. "The kinked veins at the knees and hips further increase the resistance to flow."

In fact, stress on the vein walls is doubled when you sit in a chair, and the pressure in the ankles is 250 times greater in a chair than if you sat on the floor. "It's really a matter of plumbing," says Dr. Baron.

And you can add injury to injury. Many of Dr. Baron's patients return from their overseas vacations with more than wonderful memories and slides. They get phlebitis, and not from wandering the exotic back alleys of Paris and Madrid. It's the eight-hour flight to and from that does them in. Phlebitis, a blood-clotting condition that's a frequent complication of varicose veins, is thought to be caused by pooling of blood in the veins.

Sitting may possibly have another serious complication — colon cancer. Researchers at the University of Southern California School of Medicine took a look at a group of 2,950 men with colon cancer, whom they ranked according to occupational activity levels. What they discovered was that the men in sedentary occupations—accountants, engineers and bank officers, for example—had a colon cancer risk at least 1.6 times that of men whose jobs were more active, such as longshoremen and freight handlers (*American Journal of Epidemiology,* June, 1984).

Though the scientists are far from providing firm explanations, they did speculate about the reason for their findings. Exercise, they say, appears to stimulate the colon, resulting in shortened transit time of the stool and less contact between the membranes of the colon and cancer-causing substances in the diet. Theoretically, at least, the less time you spend sitting still, the lower your risk of colon cancer.

The same holds true for the other ailments sitting flesh is heir to. Probably the smartest thing you can do if you sit a lot is not sit a lot, say the experts, who offer this compendium of good advice that starts with getting you on your feet.

Get Up and Go

"Exercise, walk, run, jump, jog, anything," urges Dr. Baron. "Anything that keeps your legs moving and your circulation going."

For varicose vein sufferers, Dr. Baron recommends something just short of perpetual motion, even if you're still sitting down. At your desk or crammed into an airline seat, you can still flex your calf muscles to get your venous "heart" pumping. "Press your feet against the floor or, on an airplane, on the seat bar. Start wiggling your toes against the floor. Get up every hour or so and walk. If you're on an airplane, walk up and down the aisles. It's a good argument for flying coach. It's a long walk," says the surgeon.

Shelley Liebman is a fitness consultant who counsels office workers in the Washington, D.C., area on the best way to stay fit behind a desk. In fact, she wrote a book on her techniques, called *Do It at Your Desk: An Office Worker's Guide to Fitness and Health* (Berkeley Press, 1984).

"My best advice for people with back problems or varicose veins is don't sit for more than an hour at a time," she says. "Get up and get a drink of water. Arrange it so your typing paper is across the room."

Ms. Randolph recommends some painless exercises to keep you pain free and limber. "Put your hands in the small of your back and arch backward," she says. "Stand intermittently."

Squatting helps stretch and lengthen leg muscles, which tend to tighten if we sit too much or break up our sedentary existence with jogging.

The squat also has an honored history. It's probably what *Homo erectus* did before he discovered a hard surface to sit on. "Even today members of primitive societies don't sit in chairs; they squat," says Robert M. Martin II, M.D., a Pasadena, California, physician. "There are a lot of Vietnamese in this country, and when you see them waiting for buses, they squat. They're using their legs as shock absorbers. When you sit on a hard surface, your shock-absorption system is destroyed. The Vietnamese don't have the kind of low back problems we have."

Posture Pointers

Forget the ramrod-stiff military cadet pose drilled into you at home and in school, says David F. Fardon, M.D., founder of the Knoxville Back Care Center in Tennessee and author of *Free Yourself from Back Pain* (Prentice-Hall, 1984). In fact, you can forget just about everything your mother ever told you about sitting still, keeping your elbows off the table and not rocking forward in your chair.

"Don't be afraid to move around in your chair," says the orthopedic surgeon. "Children know they are more comfortable if they wiggle in their chairs, but they are taught to sit still . . . Children innately know what's comfortable and good for them. They lean forward in their chairs, balancing on the front legs. Their mothers get them to stop doing it, of course, because it busts up the furniture. But it does shift the stresses off the lower back in much the same way the Balans chair from Sweden does, which has a forward-tilted seat and knee rest."

Though there's no "best" sitting posture, says Dr. Fardon, it does help to start out with your feet flat on the floor and your knees and hips at right angles to the floor and each other. Armrests can take some body weight off your spine, but resting the forearms and elbows on the desk or table can do the same thing.

Do not, under any circumstances, ever cross your legs, warn the experts. Sitting cross-legged nearly doubles the stress on your spine and tissues.

Make Adjustments

"Many people work in chairs that can be adjusted and don't know it," says Dr. Fardon. "They've never gotten under the chair and figured out what all the knobs do. They just sit in a chair they've inherited from the guy before them, who may have been taller, shorter, of entirely different dimensions."

Most good work chairs can be adjusted for height and have an adjustable backrest. In some chairs, the seat also tilts backward and forward with your body.

"Get a standing desk if you can," suggests Augustus A. White III, M.D., chief of orthopedic surgery at Boston's Beth Israel Hospital and author of *Your Aching Back: A Doctor's Guide to Relief* (Bantam Books, 1983). "If you can't get one, spend some time during the day standing. For instance, when you talk on the phone, get a long cord so you can walk around while you're speaking."

If you aren't lucky enough to have adjustable equipment, make some adjustments yourself. Roll up a towel and attach it to your backrest at the curve of your lower back to help maintain the comfortable, natural sway of your spine. Bring a small footstool to work to keep your legs raised slightly, or simply substitute a large phone book.

An air pillow or adjustable orthopedic seat can make driving more comfortable. If you can't find or afford them, substitute a towel or small pillow from home and relax your spine by draping your arms over the steering wheel, says Dr. White.

If you want to make a bigger investment to protect your back on the road, put a down payment on a car with an orthopedic seat and a suspension system that cushions the spine from the damaging effects of road vibrations.

Dr. White says he hasn't written out a prescription quite yet, "but I have a few patients who've bought cars for their well-designed seats to suit their backs. It's best to ask fellow back sufferers which brands are best."

HOW TO CHOOSE A CHAIR

"A well-constructed chair may add as much as 40 productive minutes to the working day of each productive individual," says E. R. Tichauer, Ph.D., author of *The Biomechanical Basis of Ergonomics* (Wiley-Interscience Publication).

A poorly designed chair can force you to waste that much time just trying to get comfortable.

How do you know if you have a good chair? Basically, if you ignore it. "Curiously, the most appropriate (or comfortable) chair is hardly noticed," says Dr. Marvin Dainoff of Miami University of Ohio, who is an expert in ergonomics, the science of applying human engineering to the design of the things people use. "As long as it provides proper support, it's usually ignored."

But that doesn't mean picking out a good chair is an easy operation. You've got to approach it on the order of little Goldilocks: Try as many chairs as you can until you find the one that's "just right" for your body as well as for the tasks you'll be doing in the chair.

(continued)

HOW TO CHOOSE
A CHAIR— *Continued*

The first rule of thumb: Take a test sit. "Looking at a piece of furniture in a catalog and actually seeing and experiencing it are completely different things," says Ron Sonnenleiter, a veteran furniture designer and head of Sonnenleiter Design in Rockford, Illinois. "This is especially important if you're not average size. Chairs are designed for the average."

When you're chair shopping, be on the lookout for these comfy chair musts:

• Adjustable features. A good chair moves easily up and down, has an adjustable backrest and a seat pan that tilts forward or backward to fit your needs.

• The backrest should help you maintain the natural curve of your spine, providing strong support in the small of the back. It should give gentle support across the whole back, not cut into the ribs or pelvis or interfere with the elbows.

• The seat pan should be 25 percent wider than the buttocks and end with a scroll or waterfall edge that won't cut into the thighs, which would inhibit circulation.

• An armrest, provided it doesn't get in the way of your arms and elbows while you work, takes some of the load off your spine. It also makes it easier to get in and out of the chair.

• A five-blade pedestal offers the best chair stability.

• Casters do more than give you mobility. If a chair can be pushed by leg movements, you can use it to activate the muscle pump in your legs to improve circulation.

Shrug Off Your Tension

Does life give you a *real* pain in the neck? Does tension build slowly in your shoulders during the day until they feel like they're reinforced with concrete? Have your neck and shoulders become your "tension center"?

You're not alone. Most of us do things every day—at work, at home and at play—that inject tension into the muscles of our necks and shoulders. We literally shoulder our burdens, both physical and emotional.

"I call it carrying the weight of the world on your shoulders," says Susan L. Fish, a registered physical therapist in New York City. "It's the second most common problem that I see, after low back pain."

If you're feeling a lot like Atlas these days, don't despair. You may be able to cast off your burden simply by changing some of your tension-toting habits.

"One major cause of neck and shoulder pain is a round-shouldered posture," Ms. Fish claims. "It throws our heads forward and leaves us looking down. But we tend to want to see where we're going. So we arch our heads back. Holding our heads up in that forward-jutting position puts a tremendous amount of stress on the muscles in the back of the neck and upper shoulders. And a muscle that's in a constant state of contraction can become a painful muscle.

"Part of the problem is habit. Part is genetic. Part is just generally poor posture, from the feet all the way up. For instance, large-busted women may get round-shouldered because of the weight of their breasts. In postmenopausal women, osteoporosis can contribute to it. And fatigue can cause you to be round-shouldered because people who don't get enough sleep just can't hold themselves up straight."

Slouching in your easy chair is another way to make your neck and shoulders uneasy. "If you let yourself scoot down in your chair and slouch in your lower back, you're going to go into that round-shouldered posture," says Ms. Fish. "One of the best ways to avoid that is to support your lower back.

When you sit right up on the base of your buttocks with a support in your lower back, it's hard to slouch over. Lumbar-support chairs are helpful for that reason."

Putting yourself in the driver's seat can also throw you out of alignment. "Many automobile seats are designed to allow you to slouch down," Ms. Fish points out. "Again, I recommend that my patients use back supports and sit erect. But I don't want to minimize the fact that I give all of my patients with neck and shoulder pain an individualized exercise program geared to strengthening the upper back muscles, stretching the inner chest muscles and maintaining posture where the spine is straight."

Don't Look Down

People who constantly look down at their work are going to strain the neck and shoulders, too. "After about an hour of working at my computer terminal, my shoulders and neck would begin to ache," recounts David Rosenkrantz, an engineer. "The pain would get worse as the day went on. I'd get so uncomfortable that I couldn't concentrate. I had to do something, so one day I tried raising the monitor. That alleviated most of the stiffness. It turns out that because I'm tall, I was constantly looking down to read the screen."

"It's common for typists and people who work at computers to have neck and shoulder pain," says Ms. Fish. "Typists should use a book stand to copy from, rather than laying the source flat on the desk. And computer users should have the screen at eye level," she advises. "That will keep them from constantly tiring those neck muscles."

If you're having trouble reading the fine print these days, you could be sticking your neck out. "Nearsighted people often jut their heads forward so they can see better," Ms. Fish told us. "That can also cause neck and shoulder pain. Corrective lenses should take care of it, if the person has not already developed the habit of leaning forward."

Reading in bed with your head propped up on a tower of pillows can also put a kink in your neck. Your chest, it seems, is a poor choice for a chin rest. Ms. Fish recommends using angled pillows that hold the head straight but elevate the whole upper body.

Excess Baggage

Could your shoulder bag carry the U.S. mail? Could your briefcase anchor the Queen Mary? Carrying a heavy load continuously on one side will almost certainly make your neck and shoulders cry uncle. "One day I was carrying a heavy shoulder bag when I went shopping," recalls Ellen Moser, a housewife. "Hours later I got a funny feeling in my neck. I thought it was nothing. But when I woke up the next morning it was terribly painful. So I went to the emergency room at a local hospital. The doctor who saw me figured out that the pain was from carrying the heavy shoulder bag.

"The pain lasted for about six weeks and kept me up at night. It took a long time to heal, but it eventually went away. I just made sure not to carry the shoulder bag for any length of time. And if I was going shopping, I unloaded everything except the necessities—like money."

"When you carry a heavy shoulder bag or briefcase, you wind up with your body tilted over," explains Ms. Fish. "But you hold your head upright so you can see straight. So one side of your neck is constantly contracted. The muscle never totally relaxes. If you have to carry heavy things, divide the weight evenly between both of your arms. If you must wear a shoulder bag, switch sides occasionally. And, if at all possible, try not to use one at all."

Even something as second nature as talking on the telephone can call up pain in your muscles. "Holding a telephone between your ear and your shoulder really contributes to keeping those upper shoulder muscles in a constant state of tension. People who do that habitually should get either a phone rest or a headset," Ms. Fish recommends.

To a large extent, neck and shoulder problems are side effects of 20th-century life. The causes—using a computer, talking on the telephone, carrying a briefcase—are the postures of modern man. But the problems are also related to the *pace* of modern man.

Please Release Me

"Every time something upsets you or you feel aggravated, your body tenses up," explains Dennis T. Jaffe, Ph.D., professor of psychology at Saybrook Institute in San Francisco and coauthor of *From Burnout to Balance* (McGraw-Hill, 1984). "It's part of the body's reaction to anything that's threatening. Your muscles tense up, your breathing gets shallower, you secrete adrenaline, and your whole body gets thrown into overdrive. That's what the stress response is.

"The problem is that most of the things that are upsetting to us do not require that kind of a response. It's inappropriate to respond physically even though your body is responding physically. And if you don't do something to release the muscle tension, it stays there, even after the upset is over. Your body doesn't rebound to normal.

"And so, over the course of a day, muscle tension builds up. Many people have a tendency to hold that tension in their neck and shoulders.

"Physically active people definitely have less trouble with it," Dr. Jaffe points out, "because they're out there releasing their muscles all the time. But people who are sitting all day, especially if they're hunched over, need to find ways to release the tension."

If your shoulders are nearly touching your ears, that's a clue that you're holding tension in them. "I sometimes have patients look in the mirror, then I tell them to drop their shoulders. Some people drop them about three inches," says Ms. Fish. "When they see it in the mirror, they become aware of the fact that their shoulders were almost touching their earlobes. It's really an education. Many people don't even know that they're doing it.

"I find the most beneficial thing to recommend is axial extension, or elongating the neck. To do that, look straight ahead, keeping your chin parallel to the floor. Imagine that your head is being pulled straight up. When you do axial extension, you're forced to relax the muscles in your shoulders and drop them down. The result is correct posture.

"The one thing I usually would not do," says Ms. Fish,

"is give a patient a cervical collar unless there is a neurological problem as well. If they wear a collar, they'll weaken their muscles. I don't use collars for this kind of muscle tension problem."

But there are many other things you can do to help relax those muscles. "Letting a hot shower run on the back of your neck is probably one of the most effective ways to relax the neck and shoulder muscles," says Paul J. Rosch, M.D., president of the American Institute of Stress in Yonkers, New York.

"Progressive muscle relaxation exercises are also very helpful. To do them, you progressively tense, then relax, the different muscle groups in your body. For example, you may start with your hands, then tense and relax your forearms, then your upper arms, then your shoulders and so on. That's one technique that's used by a variety of practitioners to relax muscles and reduce stress. Deep breathing seems to help, too."

Breaking the Cycle

More serious cases may benefit from professional attention. "When a muscle goes into spasm, sometimes it sets up a vicious circle," Dr. Rosch points out. "It may contract down on the nerve that carries the sensation of pain. If it does that, the nerve becomes irritated, which causes continued muscle spasm. In some instances it's possible to break that cycle by injecting an anesthetic to release the spasm. When the spasm is reduced, there's no longer any pressure on the nerve and you break the cycle. Pain-relieving, anti-inflammatory and muscle relaxant drugs can also be effective if they break the spasm/pain cycle.

"However," cautions Dr. Rosch, "if you have persistent pain that used to be relieved by simple analgesics like aspirin and no longer is, that's a sign that you should see a physician. You should also seek medical attention if you have numbness or tingling in your arms or fingers, pain down your arms, or changes in the muscle tone in your arms or hands."

"I treat a lot of this muscle spasm with electrical stimulation," says Ms. Fish. "That's the use of electricity to stop the muscle spasms. Some people use ultrasound as well. The deep heat it creates increases the circulation."

"When a muscle is tense, the flow of blood can be cut off," says Marilyn Frender, a licensed massage therapist in New York City and editor of the *American Massage Therapy Association Journal.* "Massage can increase circulation, warming the muscles and taking out tension. It can soothe and relax the muscles as well as calm the person. It's good for general body relaxation and stress reduction.

"You don't need to be an expert, either. You can help someone relax their shoulders by running your hands smoothly from the nape of the neck across the shoulders, stroking toward the heart. There are seminars available in many cities that teach self-massage and massage for couples. Or if you prefer, you can try to locate a licensed massage therapist through local medical practitioners or health clubs."

"The important thing," says Dr. Rosch, "is to recognize where the sources of stress are in your life that might be causing this."

Dr. Jaffe agrees. "Anything that's upsetting or creates conflict in your life can give you tension. It's important to look at the stress in your life and make changes. If you release the tension but keep going back into the same kind of stress, you'll just keep creating problems for yourself."

Practical
Psychology
Updates

How to Boost
Your Brainpower

Water lilies double in area every 24 hours. At the beginning of the summer there is one water lily on a lake. It takes 60 days for the lake to become covered with water lilies. On what day is the lake half covered?

How does your mind work when you read a brainteaser like this? Is it tickled pink—or tormented to tears? Is it too tired to tackle the task? Do you spend time puzzling over an answer, or lose interest if it doesn't jump right out at you? Do you logically begin counting lily pads from day one? Or, without much apparent effort, does your mind leap to the solution? If the lake is totally covered on day 60, it must be half covered on. . .why, day 59, of course. Why didn't *I* think of that?!

We all have days when our thinking is fuzzy, when our logic defies reason, when we can't for the life of us remember some name or fact that was so familiar just the day before. On days like those you might want to trade in your gray matter for a new, improved model with rechargeable batteries and a software system that lets you discover the unknown secrets of the universe in one easy lesson.

Unfortunately, we have to make do with what Mother Nature has given us. Luckily, that's usually more than adequate. But it doesn't mean we can't make better use of the brainpower we do have. Here are some ways to do just that.

Poor Posture — Poor Thinking?

Ever feel like you just can't think straight? Check to see if your posture is putting a crimp on the blood supply to your brain, says E. Fritz Schmerl, M.D., teacher of gerontology at Chabot College, Hayward, California.

"The brain needs up to 30 times more blood than other organs," Dr. Schmerl says. "But allowing your upper body to sag — with rounded shoulders, head hung over and chin jutting outward — can create kinks in the spine that squeeze the two arteries passing through the spinal column to the brain, causing an inadequate blood supply." The result? "Fuzzy thinking and forgetfulness, especially as we age," says Dr. Schmerl.

Hunched-over posture can contribute to strokelike symptoms, known as transient ischemic attacks, which are brief blackout periods. Worse yet, disturbances in the blood flow of the pinched artery might cause a buildup of fatty deposits that can cause partial blockage, according to Dr. Schmerl.

"It's important to get a head start on proper alignment while you're young," Dr. Schmerl says. "Poor posture is a hard habit to break when you're older. Be consciously on guard to prevent this process by holding yourself straight, with your head back and your chin in," he says.

Iron-Poor Intellect

The brain needs large amounts of oxygen to function effectively, and the only way it can get it is through iron-packed red blood cells, says Don M. Tucker, Ph.D., associate professor of psychology at the University of Oregon at Eugene.

Some studies show that children with iron-deficiency anemia have short attention spans and trouble learning new material. They also show that boosting iron intake reverses these problems.

And Dr. Tucker's research shows that adults can suffer from related problems with alertness and memory when their iron levels are in the "low but normal" range.

In one study, for instance, the higher the blood iron levels, the greater the word fluency. (Volunteers were asked to come up with as many words as they could that begin with "Q" and end with "L".) In another study, in adults over age 60, blood iron levels were one of the more important measures in determining whether or not the person had normal brain wave patterns.

"Getting enough oxygen to the brain is certainly part of its function, but we think iron also influences brain chemicals and pathways," Dr. Tucker says. "We know now that iron is heavily concentrated in a part of the reticular activating system. This area of the brain turns the brain on, so to speak. It maintains alertness. So we can't help but think that iron plays an important role in awareness and alertness."

Aerobic Aptitude

Exercise makes people feel good and can help lift depression. Now, researchers are finding that it also builds mental "muscles" and may postpone aging's effects on the brain.

Researchers in Utah recently found that reaction time, short-term memory and the ability to reason all greatly improved in a group of out-of-shape people aged 55 to 70 who were put on a four-month program of brisk walking. They were better able to remember sequences of numbers, for instance, or to use abstract thinking to correctly match numbers and symbols.

"I was surprised at the amount of improvement we saw," says Robert Dustman, Ph.D., of the Salt Lake City Veterans Administration Hospital. "We expected to see some results in some people, but we didn't think it would be across the board."

Aerobic exercise makes the body better at transporting oxygen to all its organs, "so we are assuming that the brain benefits by receiving more oxygen," Dr. Dustman says. Those who showed the most improvement (their scores rose by 27 percent) had walked long and hard enough to be aerobically fit.

Stay Stimulated

Mental gymnastics may do as much as physical exercise to keep our brains healthy. In fact, there's evidence that the brain may actually increase in size when it's regularly "stretched out."

Being in an environment that makes you use your brain helps keep your thinking sharp and efficient, says Marion C. Diamond, Ph.D., a professor in the University of California's department of physiology and anatomy. Boredom, on the other hand, can cause restlessness, depression and a lack of fulfillment, all of which can interfere with thinking at your best.

Dr. Diamond has studied the effects of an enriched environment on the brain cells of young rats. After the rats had spent a month in a roomy cage that included playmates and plenty of gizmos to fiddle around with, their brains actually showed increased thickness in the outer layers of the cerebral cortex, which represents an increase in the dendrites. "The rats' brains became heavier and more chemically active," Dr. Diamond says. The rats also went on to run a maze better than those that hadn't been in the enriched environment. "So they became better learners, too," she says. "I've seen the same results raising my children and teaching my students. The greater the exposure, the more adaptable they are to facing other problems."

Keeping yourself stimulated should be a lifetime pursuit, Dr. Diamond says. "Keep dreaming and satisfying those dreams. Keep looking forward, and each time you come to a lull, decide what new thing you want to do with your life, the new people you want to meet, how you're going to help people. Make changes, and make each change a new beginning."

Stock Up on Lecithin

Many of the foods touted as "brain foods"—fish, for instance, and liver and eggs—contain choline, a substance researchers are finding really can help preserve the brain's ability to reason, learn and remember.

For instance, researchers at Ohio State University recently found that mice fed a diet heavy in choline-rich lecithin, or one of lecithin's "brain-active" ingredients, phosphatidylcholine, had much better memory retention than mice on regular diets. They took much longer to go into a back room in their cages where they had received a mild electric shock, meaning they hadn't forgotten their unpleasant experience.

What's more, their brain cells, examined under a microscope, showed fewer of the expected signs of aging, says Ronald Mervis, Ph.D., of Ohio State University's Brain Aging and Neuronal Plasticity Research Group.

"Normally, as the brain ages, its cell membranes become

more rigid with fatty deposits and lose their ability to take in and release brain chemicals and to relay messages," Dr. Mervis says. This can cause memory loss and confused thinking.

But a lecithin-rich diet seems to repress or delay this membrane hardening.

"Despite the differences between mice and men, there are, nevertheless, remarkable similarities in the structure of their nerve cells," says Dr. Mervis. "I believe lecithin could help to repress or delay similar problems in man, although we have yet to verify that."

"B" Smart

The brain seems to have a special need for the B vitamins. Memory loss, disorientation, hallucination, depression, lack of coordination and personality changes can occur with B-complex deficiencies.

Alcoholics, for instance, who sometimes develop thiamine (vitamin B_1) deficiencies, have problems with short-term memory. They may remember in detail that little café in Paris 20 years ago, but not what they had for supper the previous night. Thiamine-deficient mice have trouble balancing on a tightrope, a skill that's normally a snap for them.

B_{12} deficiencies have been linked with poor memory and an inability to concentrate. And recently, researchers at the University of New Mexico School of Medicine in Albuquerque found that people age 60 or older with even a mild B_{12} deficiency had poor memories and abstract thinking skills. (They had trouble repeating a short story and matching symbols with numbers.) "I think it's likely that in older people subclinical deficiencies can indeed lead to less-than-optimal mental performance," says James Goodwin, M.D., one of the study's researchers.

Thiamine is needed to produce and use one of the brain's major chemical messengers, acetylcholine, says Gary E. Gibson, Ph.D., a thiamine researcher at the Cornell-Burke Rehabilitation Hospital, White Plains, New York. And since the B-complex vitamins are chemically related and may perform some similar functions, it's possible that others are also involved in brain chemical actions, Dr. Gibson says.

Think You Can

Telling yourself you just weren't born smart, that you can never remember things, or that you're too old to learn are good ways to sabotage your true intellectual potential, say David Lewis, Ph.D., and James Greene, authors of *Thinking Better* (Rawson, Wade Publishers, 1962). Such negative thoughts "put your brain behind bars." They keep you from pursuing knowledge and learning better ways to remember. They can push you into a mental rut as you age.

Feeling good about your ability to learn is important to intellectual functioning, and it's one of the first things to be tackled at Mankind Research Unlimited, a Silver Spring, Maryland, "superlearning" center that has turned high school dropouts into gifted learners and blind people into computer programmers.

"We tell people who don't think they can learn that they really have a lot more brain than they think, and that they can learn to use more of it than they ever thought possible," says director Carl Schleicher, Ph.D.

His learning program uses a number of different techniques —listening to stately baroque music, visualizing a quiet, private getaway place for thinking, and breathing deeply to create an aura of relaxed awareness. Then the student receives suggestions—that he *will* do better, that he *can* learn. He begins to picture himself doing that successfully, and his successes in real life are praised. He may also use creative imagery to bolster a sagging self-image. An insecure scientist might practice imagining himself in the role of a successful professional in his own field—Albert Einstein, let's say, or if he prefers a neater-looking appearance, Robert Oppenheimer.

"Limits on learning are self-imposed," Dr. Schleicher says. Make the sky your limit by keeping your thinking powers fit.

Enjoy a Happy Baby

Some people seem to believe that a baby is just a little blob of protoplasm with all the intelligence and complexity of a goldfish. How to make it happy? Easy. Until the little blob gets older, all it requires is a dry bottom, a full tummy and a warm blanket.

Sensitive mothers know—probably have always known—that these ideas are dead wrong, but perhaps not even mothers can guess just *how* wrong. Research of the last decade has revealed that the infant human knows more, does more and is more than anyone ever imagined.

"A baby is already a person with unique characteristics, a complex personality and all the emotions that grownups have," says Alvin N. Eden, M.D., chairman and director of the department of pediatrics at Wyckoff Heights Hospital in Brooklyn and author of *Positive Parenting* (New American Library, 1982). "Even new infants can hear, see, respond to their surroundings and interact with adults far better than most people realize."

Indeed, in the last ten years researchers have discovered that immediately after birth a baby can see a face at close range, and only hours later can deliberately choose to focus on patterns instead of solid colors. They've shown that a newborn can distinguish odors, tastes and sounds of varying volume, length, rhythm and pitch (even sounds only one note apart). There are even reports that an infant can detect the difference between a recording of his own cries and those of another baby.

And, perhaps most significant of all, studies show that a baby is capable of learning from the time of birth. Some evidence even suggests that newborns may be learning how to talk months before they actually speak. Slow-motion analysis of sound movies has revealed that one-day-old infants move their bodies in precise rhythms in perfect sync with adult speech patterns.

All of which means that a baby, like any other complicated and aware creature, needs more than simple sustenance to be happy. Fortunately, a lot of pediatricians and astute parents know (and researchers have confirmed) what many of these basic requirements are. Here are some of the most important.

Tactile Magic

Almost as nourishing for baby as mother's milk and twice as mysterious is mother's touch. So says a long line of scientific studies from around the world. The research suggests that babies who get a lot of extra holding and caressing (especially in the first months after birth) cry less, smile more and generally have more satisfying relationships with their mothers. But even more compelling are the studies showing that infants who aren't touched enough simply don't grow properly.

The latest word on this touch/growth connection comes from researchers Tiffany Fields, Ph.D., of the University of Miami Medical School, and Saul Schanberg, M.D., of Duke University Medical Center in Durham, North Carolina, and his colleagues. For ten days the researchers gave daily massages to premature infants who were in intensive care. Compared with preemies who weren't massaged, these infants gained 47 percent more weight each day, showed more mature infant behavior, appeared more active and alert, and were discharged from the hospital an average of six days earlier.

Dr. Schanberg speculates that the slowed growth of babies deprived of mother's touch is a kind of survival mechanism. He bases this observation on his years of studying the behavior of rats and their pups. The absence of the mother is life-threatening, he says, and a pup senses this threat when it isn't touched. It then shifts its energy from growing to maintaining the body as is. Human infants, he maintains, may react precisely the same way.

But how much contact is enough? Can too much cuddling spoil a baby? According to Mary D. Salter Ainsworth, Ph.D., professor of psychology at the University of Virginia in Charlottesville, the answer is no. When she conducted a year-long study of 26 infants and their mothers, she discovered that babies who were most frequently held closely cried less—even when left alone. Apparently the infants who got the most hugs also felt independent enough to do without them occasionally.

"It's nearly impossible," says Dr. Ainsworth, "to give a baby too much close bodily contact in the first few months."

Modulated Sound

As every parent knows, babies respond to sound—and thus we have a proliferation of rattles, music boxes and musical mobiles. But that's only half the story. Babies respond to particular sounds in particular ways and are happiest when they're surrounded by the right ones.

We now know, for example, that rhythmic sounds of low pitch and a slow pace (like a heartbeat) soothe babies—in fact, soothe them better than silence. In one study, 24 newborns were exposed to a beating metronome, a recording of a heartbeat, a lullaby being sung and no sound at all. The infants cried less, moved less, had lower heart rates and breathed more regularly when they heard the rhythmic sounds. A similar study showed that even a continuous sound, like a steady tone, could soothe babies better than silence.

But of all sounds, nothing seems to gratify infants like the human voice—especially the higher-pitched female voice. Research suggests that babies just days old react more to voices and voicelike sound than to other noises. Infants, apparently, are tuned into sound frequencies in the range of human speech.

"Babies are social and responsive beings," says Dr. Eden, "and therefore benefit from hearing your voice. They may not understand the meaning of your words, but they do understand and respond to your tone of voice."

For infants, however, there is such a thing as too much sound. In a recent study, Theodore D. Wachs, Ph.D., professor of psychology at Purdue University, found that infants in homes with high noise levels showed delays in development. Dr. Wachs concludes, "Excessive household noise (from things like TVs, radios and stereos) may delay cognitive growth in infants as young as seven months and lead later to significant behavioral and language deficits."

And how much noise is too much? "If you're in a room with a baby and you can't hear him when he makes sounds," says Dr. Wachs, "there's probably too much noise."

The Moving Experience

Mothers know this: Rocking quiets little hearts. But scientists know this: Almost any kind of dramatic movement—rocking or otherwise—can force significant changes in an infant.

Research shows that moving a baby about—by walking him, swaying with him, picking him up or whatever—can calm his mood and maybe even stimulate his development.

Perhaps the most dramatic demonstration of the soothing power of movement is a study conducted by Anneliese Korner, Ph.D., and her colleagues at Stanford University School of Medicine. They wanted to see which method of soothing worked best on 40 newborns. They tried simply holding the babies in the nursing position, talking to them, touching them without picking them up, lifting them to the shoulder with their heads supported and several other strategies. The clear winner: lifting the infants to the shoulder, the method involving the most movement.

"When the babies were picked up and moved to the shoulder," says Dr. Korner, "they not only stopped crying but opened their eyes and looked around." The most rapid and drastic changes in the babies' positions seemed to get the best results.

Corroborating evidence for Dr. Korner's study comes from McGill University in Montreal. There researchers found that carrying 4- to 12-week-old babies around when they're asleep or content—as well as when they're feeding or crying—reduces total crying time by 25 to 45 percent.

A Trusting Soul

Does your baby trust you? The traditional answer is that adults trust; babies just eat and sleep. But a new generation of baby experts (including many parents) says that babies are emotionally sophisticated from the moment of birth and that their feelings of trust are key to their future mental health.

Dr. Eden says that trusting infants feel that their world is reliable, that their needs will be met. And other authorities say that thwarting such feelings can cause emotional problems that persist for years—frustration, stress, blunted sensitivity and more. Some experts even claim that an infant's mistrust can be the source of a lifelong pessimism.

Trusting infants, says Dr. Eden, come from accepting parents, parents who see infants as benign and vulnerable people whose cries signal legitimate needs. "If you believe in and accept the concept that your little girl is dependent and immature and that your role as parent is to meet her needs," Dr. Eden says, "the rest is easy."

Distrustful babies, on the other hand, come from parents who don't respond well to infants' needs because they think babies are naturally selfish and demanding.

"It is sad but true," says Dr. Eden, "that many parents are sure that their babies are devious, cunning and manipulative, that giving in to their babies' needs will lead to spoiling. But attending promptly and completely to a baby's desires leads to his contentment, not unacceptable behavior."

Some Clean Air

Although many adults are bothered by cigarette smoke, is it safe to assume that babies are too young to notice when their parents puff away? Not according to a group of French researchers.

Recently they questioned the mothers of 253 infants and discovered that 91 percent of the infants whose fathers smoked more than 20 cigarettes daily were colicky. Just 57 percent of babies who had mothers who smoked (and had nonsmoking fathers) were colicky. And only 32 percent of babies with nonsmoking parents had colic regularly. The researchers concluded that babies' taste and smell systems are just too sensitive to withstand the smoke and odor of tobacco (*British Medical Journal,* September 15, 1984).

Apparently, smoke-free air is another minimum daily requirement for happy babies.

A New, Natural
Body Normalizer

Delores Borough's migraine headaches had been ruining her weekends for three years. "They'd often come on a Saturday morning, which meant I'd either spend a day or two in bed or force myself to do things with my family even though I felt awful," the Topeka, Kansas, homemaker says. What's more, they were getting worse, and she was afraid she'd soon need stronger pain medication.

Luckily, that's all history. Now, when Mrs. Borough feels a migraine coming on, she quickly sits down, closes her eyes and imagines she's stretched out on a blissful tropical beach. The sun is shining away, focusing its radiating warmth right on her hands.

In less than a minute the temperature of her hands does begin to rise—usually several degrees—and her pending headache disappears. She may continue to warm her hands this way every half hour or so until she can feel that the migraine is no longer a threat.

Warming your *hands* to prevent a *headache*? It might sound like a new twist to the old snake-oil cure, but it's worked for people around the country. "Yes, it all sounded pretty far-out to me, too," Mrs. Borough admits, "until I saw for myself that I *could* do it and that my headaches *had* gone away."

Ten or 15 years ago, such a mind-over-body feat would have been considered the realm of yogis and other mystics, possibly, but certainly not Midwestern housewives. Today, though, this temperature biofeedback technique is becoming positively mainstream.

Mrs. Borough learned her skills at the Menninger Foundation in Topeka, which has pioneered research in this area. Other major medical facilities around the country, including Harvard, Yale, Johns Hopkins and the Mayo Clinic, are using temperature control of the hands and other body parts in their biofeedback or stress-reduction programs.

Most often treated with this technique are circulatory-related problems like migraines, high blood pressure and Raynaud's disease, in which the arteries in the hands clamp shut. But hand warming has also worked to relieve arthritis, angina, irritable bowel syndrome, diabetes, menopausal problems and impotence.

"These aren't illnesses in the infectious-disease sense," says Elmer E. Green, Ph.D., founder of the Menninger Foundation's Biofeedback and Psychophysiology Center. "They're chronic conditions with a strong psychosomatic link. And if we can make ourselves sick this way, we can use our minds to make ourselves well again."

Dr. Green was studying body changes during autogenic training (a learned relaxation technique) when he discovered by chance that hand warming could banish a migraine.

"During autogenic training, people often reported that their hands felt warmer," Dr. Green says. "We wanted to find out if indeed this was true, and if people could make their hands warm just by thinking about it."

One of his first subjects happened to be a woman who had suffered from migraines for years. When she began doing the autogenic training hand-warming exercises, her headaches suddenly vanished. "Another woman never had a headache again until the day she died 11 years later," Dr. Green says. And it's not unusual for people who complete Menninger's migraine headache training program to get similar results, Dr. Green says.

Short-Circuits the Stress Response

Hand warming works by counteracting the body's reaction to stress, Dr. Green says.

Under real or imagined stress, the body's autonomic, or automatic, nervous system takes over. Muscles tense, arteries to the hands and feet constrict (producing that cold, clammy feeling), blood pressure rises, and heart and breathing rates increase. Body chemistry changes; there's more adrenaline in the blood, for instance. What is happening is that we're preparing physically for fight or flight, says Steven Fahrion, Ph.D., director of Menninger's hypertension program.

"This would be fine if you were being chased by a hungry

bear," Dr. Fahrion says. "But we unconsciously react physically to many situations in everyday life as though they are life-threatening, and this inevitably hurts us by creating stress-related ailments."

But biofeedback training helps your conscious mind become aware of your body's physical response to stress, so you can learn to recognize the subtle internal cues that tell you whether you are tense or relaxed. And then, as Dr. Green puts it, you can learn to "go with" the feeling of relaxation. "What we're doing is teaching people to recognize the body sensations of both stress and relaxation, and to turn on the relaxation sensations at will," he says.

Hand warming can be used to induce this relaxed state, although it's most often used in conjunction with general relaxation and targeted to specific areas. It's actually a fairly easy skill to learn. Still, most people require 12 to 15 lessons to master the technique.

What you're really learning is to consciously relax the muscles in the walls of the blood vessels in your hands so that the arteries expand, blood rushes in, and the area is warmed.

It's much different from warming your hands outwardly— by putting them in hot water, for instance. That, too, dilates the blood vessels of the hands, but it won't help produce the other physical relaxation responses usually needed to stop your headache.

So How Do You Do It?

The actual mechanics of hand warming are pretty straightforward. Many biofeedback clinics have their own variations on this procedure set up by the Menninger Foundation.

First, a temperature biofeedback machine is attached to a finger of the dominant hand. (You can use a thermometer taped to your finger, or a liquid-crystal ring whose color display indicates skin temperature changes.)

Then you learn to relax your hands and entire body by silently repeating autogenic training phrases, such as "I feel quite quiet," "My arms and hands are heavy and warm," "I can feel the warmth flowing down my arms into my hands," and "My thoughts are turned inward and I am serene."

After about 20 minutes of this, you look at the temperature changes that have been recorded and then write down a short summary of your body feelings, emotions and thoughts during the session. "This is to teach you to perceive the body changes you are experiencing without always having to rely on a machine," Dr. Green says.

After about a week of twice-daily, at-home practice with a biofeedback machine, you begin to replace these phrases with your own personal visualizations relating to temperature control. Like Mrs. Borough, many people imagine lying on a beach, perhaps even burying their hands in the warm sand. "You might also imagine holding a hot, boiled egg or plunging your hands into hot, soapy water," Dr. Green says.

But eventually even this visualization becomes less and less necessary, and the control of hand temperature "is reduced to turning on an almost indescribable sensation which brings about vascular relaxation in a minute or two," Dr. Green says.

But what does all this have to do with a migraine headache?

Migraines start with a constriction of the carotid arteries, which supply blood to the brain, explains Jack Hartje, Ph.D., a University of North Florida biofeedback professor and a former migraine sufferer himself. "Certain foods, stress or temperature changes can trigger this response. When the brain senses it isn't getting enough blood, it releases neurochemicals that, in migraine sufferers, cause a painful overdilation of these arteries."

Doing hand warming when you first sense the constriction may prevent this whole sequence of events, Dr. Hartje says.

Leg Warming, Too

The Menninger Foundation's hypertension program combines both hand *and* leg warming for a success rate that's hard to beat.

"Seventy percent of our patients are able to get off their medication completely, and to get their blood pressure down an average of 10 to 15 points below their initial reading with medication," Dr. Fahrion says. In fact, those taking the most drugs initially seem to do best on the program, perhaps because they are more motivated. And these aren't just mild hypertensives.

"We do have some who want to prevent high blood pressure, but I'd say the average unmedicated blood pressure of our patients would be about 180/110," Dr. Fahrion says.

Just like migraine headaches, most forms of high blood pressure are associated with vascular constriction caused by stress. (In fact, before blood pressure medicines were available, about the only way doctors could relieve constriction was by cutting certain nerves to the arms and legs. On occasion this worked so well people would faint from the effects.)

"Hand warming relieves some of this constriction, but the biggest blood pressure drop comes from the increased flow to the lower half of the body," Dr. Fahrion says. Foot warming can take several additional weeks of practice, though.

Jerry Hutchison, a University of Kansas administrator and faculty member, completed the foundation's blood pressure program two years ago. "My doctor had read about it and wanted to see if it really worked," he says.

In four months, Hutchison had learned to raise the temperature of both his hands and feet during the cold winter months, sometimes by up to 20 degrees. He was also able to stop taking all his blood pressure drugs. "And the fatigue and dull headaches I'd occasionally had went away, too.

"It's hard to explain it, but after you've done it again and again you begin to be able to key in on the feeling that makes the temperature go up," he says. "At first it's just an observation, but then it becomes an internal technique." Hutchison's blood pressure has remained at the same level as when he left the program, about 130/75. "Two years ago," he says, "I would not have believed your mind could really affect your body this way. Now I believe."

Hand-Warming Lifesaver

Hand warming made desperate sense to Chris Berman, who suffers from Raynaud's disease, a condition in which the arteries of the hand constrict for no known reason.

"My hands would actually turn blue from the wrist down," the Washington, D.C., intensive care nurse says. "I had angina-like pain in them, my fingernails were peeling off and I had dark spots where the tissue was dying. I was afraid I would lose my fingers."

Medication to keep her hand arteries open lowered her blood pressure so much she was afraid to drive. Doctors were considering several alternatives (even the radical procedure of severing nerves to her hands) when she came across information on hand warming.

"I knew immediately it was something I had to try," she says. "At first it took me about half an hour to be able to warm them up, but now I can do it while I'm sitting at a stop light. I actually envision the arteries opening up and the blood flowing into my hands."

Diabetics Helped, Too

Diabetics often develop painful and life-threatening circulation problems in their limbs because their disease causes atherosclerosis, says Daniel Cox, Ph.D., an associate professor in the department of behavioral medicine at the University of Virginia Medical School, Charlottesville.

"Although so far we've only taught a few diabetics to increase the circulation in their hands and feet, the results are very promising," Dr. Cox says. "All of them have been able to do this, and it's meant their leg spasms improve, they can walk longer and longer distances without pain, and their risks of eventually requiring amputation are probably less. What we'd like to do is to be able to provide diabetics with an alternative to vascular surgery."

People who have arthritis, menstrual cramps or hot flashes can also benefit from hand warming, says Keith Sedlacek, M.D., adjunct professor at the City College of New York and director of the Stress Regulation Institute.

"Older people often have problems associated with poor circulation in their arms and legs," Dr. Sedlacek says. "Hand and foot warming increases oxygen and lubrication in the joints, and can reduce swelling. They can move with less pain, which encourages them to exercise more. And in another few years we should have enough evidence to see if it's slowed the progress of their disease, as I suspect it does."

Women experiencing hot flashes as a result of menopause can actually learn to stabilize their capillaries and avert an episode, Dr. Sedlacek says. "Our patients who are skilled at this report 50 to 80 percent fewer hot flashes without needing further hormone treatment." Hand and foot warming also relieves menstrual cramps in about half the women he sees. Some go on to learn vaginal warming, which sometimes does the trick.

There is one side effect of hand or foot warming.

"We call it 'the enabling effect,' " Dr. Green says. "When people realize that these normally involuntary processes of the body can be controlled, they get a feeling of self-mastery that extends to other areas of their life. It's amazing how many people we treat have wanted to go on a diet, but didn't do it until they learned to warm their hands. Then they realized they have the body mastery to do that, too."

The implications of this go far beyond what most people can imagine, Dr. Green says. "The point is that medicine is going to have to change. The treatment is going to have to involve the mind of the patient. Yes, this puts a responsibility on patients, but it also gives them power."

Puts it right into their own hands, you might say.

"At the Count of 3, You Will Feel Fine!"

Like alchemy and astrology, the practice of hypnosis once belonged to the world of the occult. But then, so did medicine.

Today, numerous medical schools teach hypnosis, and a handful of doctors, dentists and psychologists are board-certified to practice it.

Although hypnosis has been used successfully to treat such things as phobias and bad habits, its most significant role has been in the treatment of pain. Doctors first used it as an anesthetic in the 1840s, and they still use it for that purpose today. In cases where chemical anesthesia is undesirable—in childbirth, or when the patient has an allergy to anesthetics—

hypnosis has proved itself to be not only effective but also inexpensive, safe and virtually free of side effects in patients able to enter profound hypnosis.

"Hypnosis is very, very good at pain control," says Eugene E. Levitt, Ph.D., secretary-treasurer of the American Board of Psychological Hypnosis and a professor at the Indiana University School of Medicine.

"That is one of its outstanding applied uses, particularly in pain due to clear-cut bodily pathology [disease]," adds Martin Orne, M.D., Ph.D., director of the unit for experimental psychiatry at the Institute of Pennsylvania Hospital. "For people who have the ability to respond well, hypnosis is one of the few effective ways of providing pain relief over a long period of time without risk."

Think "Cool and Calm"

Doctors have used hypnosis to treat many kinds of pain. In New Orleans, Dabney Ewin, M.D., a surgeon and psychiatrist who teaches hypnosis at Tulane University, uses it to treat patients with widespread third-degree burns. He's found that if he can hypnotize a burn victim within two hours after the accident, he can prevent much of the inflammation, pain and skin damage that usually results.

"In a severe burn," Dr. Ewin explains, "two things happen. There is the heat damage to the outside of the skin, and there is the inflammatory reaction from the inside, which comes as a response to the patient's fear. If I can hypnotize him into believing that he is cool and comfortable, I can turn off that response and stop the inflammation."

Others have had similar positive results. Doctors from three Minnesota children's hospitals have taught a form of self-hypnosis, "relaxation-mental imagery," to children. Of headache patients, 70 percent got relief from pain. Of 36 children with other kinds of pain, 19 got complete relief and others got partial relief (*Developmental and Behavioral Pediatrics,* February, 1984).

Obstetricians from Staten Island Hospital and Downstate Medical Center in New York have been teaching young mothers how to relax during delivery by repeating the thoughts,

"You will be calm, confident and brave. You will experience pressure and exertion but no pain. You will recover quickly and comfortably," and other suggestions.

Doctors now use hypnosis in cancer wards, according to Dr. Levitt, and there's evidence that it is effective. "The data are clear that when you introduce hypnosis techniques in a terminal cancer ward, you will see the demand for painkillers such as Demerol go down," he asserts.

Dentists often use hypnosis for patients who don't want procaine, usually with great success. Doctors have also used hypnosis to help people who suffer from migraine headaches, shingles, tinnitus, arthritis and low back pain.

Before he can treat pain, a hypnotist has to put his patient into a relaxed state. He can use a variety of induction techniques. Typically, he will speak to the patient in a gentle, rhythmic voice. He might ask the patient to close his eyes. Then, using his voice and suggesting visual images, he will soothe the patient into a state of complete relaxation.

"I ask him to visualize a stairway," one hypnotist told us. "I ask him to walk down the stairs with me, one step at a time, while I count from 20 to 1. With each step, I tell the patient that he is becoming more and more relaxed, and that by the time we reach the bottom of the stairs, his conscious mind will be asleep."

If all goes well (and it may not in the first or even the second session), the patient will slip into a hypnotic trance. Being under a trance, doctors say, is like being absorbed in a book or a film, only more so. It is a state of focused awareness and of intense concentration. In a trance, the right hemisphere of the brain is thought to become dominant, says Helen Crawford, Ph.D., of the University of Wyoming, who chairs the American Psychological Association's division on psychological hypnosis. This is associated with the nonanalytical, imaginative side of the brain, and is the one more open to suggestion.

The trance is not, however, the "zombie state" that many people imagine. "People think that in a trance a person will do anything that the hypnotist wants him to do. None of that happens in real hypnosis," says Jeanine LaBaw, Psy.D., of

Denver, who works with hypnosis and pain. "You totally maintain your own control. You won't do anything immoral. You don't take your clothes off and cluck like a chicken, unless you happen to like being the life of the party."

Once people enter a trance, a hypnotherapist enables them, in a sense, to imagine their pain away. By suggesting mental pictures at a time when the mind is especially receptive to them, the hypnotherapist can attach pain to an image and then move that image from one body part to another, or even push it out of the body. Says Daniel Kohen, M.D., associate director of behavioral pediatrics at the Minneapolis Children's Medical Center, "The active ingredient in hypnosis is imagery."

Imagery helped one man overcome back pain, for example. "One of my patients, a 45-year-old executive named Henry, suffered from severe back pain," says David E. Bresler, Ph.D., author of *Free Yourself from Pain* (Simon and Schuster, 1979). "But through symptom substitution [a mental technique for shifting pain from one place to another], he was able to move that pain from his back down to the bottoms of his feet." Eventually he was able to rid himself of his pain whenever it recurred by "walking it away." He imagined the pain leaving his body "and scattering on the ground as he walked along."

A very common technique called glove anesthesia has been used to reduce labor pain. An obstetrician might lead his patient to believe that her hand is numb by telling her under hypnosis that it's made of wood or stone or that it's a thick, woolly glove. He can then ask her, through symptom substitution, to transfer that numbness to her abdomen. After several sessions prior to birth, she will have learned to numb her belly simply by saying the word *belly.*

The possibilities are endless. "I once worked with a woman with tinnitus [a chronic, sometimes painful, ringing in the ears]," says Dr. Crawford. "Under hypnosis, I suggested that the noise in her head was like the noise of a car. She was taught that every time she felt an attack coming, she should push that car farther down the road, away from her, until she couldn't see it anymore. The noise didn't go away completely, but she learned to make it more bearable."

"Fist therapy" also helps some people. Dr. Orne asks his

patients to imagine capturing all of their pain in their fist. The tighter the fist, he says, the more pain it holds. When the pain is totally in that fist, they can throw it away and not have it come back for several hours.

The Ultimate Bedside Manner

While these techniques show *how* hypnosis works, they don't explain *why* it works. Assuming that there is no hocus-pocus involved, on what level of mind or body does hypnosis work?

One theory is that hypnosis, in a powerful way, distracts us from pain. "The explanation for suggested anesthesia," says Dr. Orne, "must probably be sought in the profound effect hypnosis may exert on selective attention." In other words, we can use the hypnotic state to focus all of our attention away from the pain.

"In experiments with cats," Dr. Orne relates, "it has been shown that the animal won't hear a clicking noise, which it normally hears, if it's hungry and we put a mouse in front of it." People can "choose to see or not to see" their pain better, he says. He also thinks that hypnosis can work by relaxing those in pain, diminishing their fear of pain.

Another theory is that during hypnosis the brain releases natural opiatelike painkillers called endorphins. This theory is espoused by Paul Sacerdote, M.D., a New York psychiatrist and oncologist who has had great success treating cancer pain.

Others believe that hypnosis acts through the emotions. Theodore X. Barber, Ph.D., a Massachusetts psychologist, thinks the success of hypnosis depends on the rapport that the doctor establishes with the person whom he or she hypnotizes. Hypnosis, he suggests, is the ultimate bedside manner, one in which doctor/patient affection pushes aside the loneliness, anxiety and tension that make pain so much worse.

At the heart of hypnosis, says Dr. Barber, is the principle that pain fluctuates depending upon the way we perceive it. "Since the interpretation of pain sensations is such an important part of the total pain experience, hypnosuggestive procedures can play an important role in pain control," he writes (*Handbook of Clinical Health Psychology,* Plenum Press, 1982).

Are You a Good Candidate?

But, supposing that hypnosis works, does that mean it will work for everyone? The question, "Who is hypnotizable?" is very much debated among researchers. The consensus is that there are a few people who can be hypnotized so deeply that they could undergo open-heart surgery without chemical anesthesia. At the other extreme are people who can't be hypnotized. Most people, however, can be hypnotized to a certain degree.

"Almost anyone can get into a trance state," says Dr. LaBaw. "If you're motivated and work on it, then you can do it. I have been using hypnosis in my practice for 14 years. In that time, only one or two people weren't hypnotizable."

But not all subjects are created equal. The better you are at letting your imagination run loose, it seems, the better your chances of being hypnotized. "The main thing is the imagination," says Ernest Hilgard, Ph.D., a Stanford University professor and a pioneer in this field. "It means having the ability to believe that you are in a nice warm pool in the South Pacific instead of sitting in a dentist's chair having your teeth drilled."

Because imagination is so big a part of their lives, children have been found to be highly hypnotizable. "We know that children whose parents read them stories are likely to be good candidates for hypnosis. By age 12, some people lose a lot of their ability to be hypnotized—a phenomenon not fully understood," says Dr. Crawford.

Dr. Barber suggests this instant "litmus test" to find out if a person is highly hypnotizable. "Ask someone to close her eyes and to imagine that she is holding a baby. Ask her to smell the baby, to feel the baby, to listen to the baby for a short while. Then tell her to open her eyes and *see* the baby. If she really sees the baby, she's a good candidate for hypnosis."

Then there are those for whom hypnosis represents the last resort for pain relief. The fact that they often focus all of their hope and attention on the doctor makes them more sensitive to trance induction. "Motivation is as important as hypnotic responsiveness in predicting the patient's ability to derive pain relief," says Dr. Orne.

But can people learn how to hypnotize themselves so that they can slip into a trance whenever pain occurs, without needing the reassuring presence of a hypnotherapist? Every doctor we spoke to said yes to this question.

Self-hypnosis, which calls on the patient to say the words of induction to himself, is effective against pain in part because it offers empowerment, doctors say. It gives patients a tool with which they can fight their pain actively. In doing so, self-hypnosis reduces the sense of helplessness that is known to make pain seem worse than it might necessarily be. "All good hypnotists teach self-hypnosis," says Dr. Hilgard.

In fact, some doctors don't even want their patients to listen to cassette tapes of their sessions when they get home, because it delays self-hypnosis. "We seldom use tapes," says Dr. LaBaw. "Using a tape is passive. People learn faster if they play an active role."

Be Your Own Therapist

You're the last one to squeeze aboard a crowded elevator, but as you begin the slow descent you realize somebody behind you wishes you'd waited for the next one. Whoever is back there is digging a blunt object very firmly and painfully into the small of your back. You're too embarrassed to make a scene, so you just stand there thinking, "I can't believe this! Who *is* that inconsiderate moron back there?"

Finally the elevator touches down on the ground floor and you step off, whirling around quickly to deliver the dirtiest look you can muster. And there stands a white-haired, sweet-faced blind lady, tottering out of the elevator on her cane. Almost instantly, your feelings change to shame and sadness, and you offer her your arm.

It's a story psychotherapist Robert Reitman, Ph.D., likes to tell to illustrate a profoundly simple point: What you *think* determines how you *feel*. If you want to change your feelings about something, it's almost impossible to simply decide not to feel sad, for instance. But you *can* change your thoughts, and more often than not your feelings will follow.

And that, in brief, is the fundamental insight behind a school of psychotherapy that's being used with great success to treat depression, anxiety, phobias, drug abuse and other problems that rob life of joy. "Cognitive therapy" is named after its primary subject—your cognitions, or thoughts. A therapist using this approach won't spend a lot of time digging around in the psychic murk of your childhood experiences or dredging up buried associations (a process that can take years, cost a small fortune and produce only questionable results). Instead, cognitive therapists operate in the present, locating and reshaping the thought patterns that are making you anxious, sad, depressed or drug dependent.

Depression: A Thinking Disorder

The technique grew out of the work of Aaron Beck, M.D., a psychiatrist at the University of Pennsylvania who set out during the 1950s to show that Freud was right when he concluded that depression was a disorder caused by turning anger inward. He concluded, after years of study, that Freud was wrong. "I discovered that in their dreams and early memories and in projective tests, depressed people see themselves as 'losers'—deprived, frustrated, rejected, humiliated or punished in some way," Dr. Beck has written. "The psychological 'cause' of depression did not appear to be buried deep in the unconscious but was related to this type of mistaken thinking."

Depression, in short, is a *thinking* disorder. In fact, depression remains a puzzle and a paradox—since it runs directly counter to the human drive for survival—only until you examine a depressed person's thoughts, says Gary Emery, Ph.D., a former student of Dr. Beck's and author of *A New Beginning* (Touchstone, 1981). A depressed housewife who feels so overwhelmed by her problems she stops trying to solve them, or can't seem to concentrate on anything except her own flaws, presents a psychological enigma until you discover that she thinks of herself as incompetent, worthless and unlikeable. The way to put her back on the road to wellness, Dr. Beck maintains, is by "changing (her) errors in thinking, rather than by concentrating on (her) depressed mood."

An interesting theory, but does it work? "Cognitive therapy has become reputable among professionals very quickly because about 12 studies so far have shown it's as effective or more effective than drugs for depression," Dr. Emery claims. One recent study at Washington University in St. Louis found that patients treated with cognitive therapy for three months responded just as well as patients treated with tricyclic antidepressants (TCAs), the most commonly prescribed antidepressant drugs. But therapy had one big advantage, observes study leader George Murphy, M.D.: It "has no unpleasant side effects and is absolutely nonfattening."

Faulty Thinking

In many ways, Dr. Emery points out, the notion that emotional problems are caused by faulty thinking isn't new at all, having been recognized a long time ago by early Greek philosophers. Cognitive therapy is "new" in that it has examined and spelled out these thinking errors in greater detail and has developed tools and techniques to alter them.

What are the thinking errors that plague the depressed? Typically, they run along lines like these:

Exaggerating ● "I just can't get myself to do any work around the house—my whole marriage is falling apart." You wildly overestimate the size of your problems at the same time you underestimate your ability to deal with them. You jump to conclusions without any evidence and erroneously believe your conclusions are correct.

Ignoring the Positive ● "Sure, the dinner party went all right, but I burned the toast points." You tend to be impressed by and remember only negative events, or view completely positive events in a negative way, often as a way of "proving" the correctness of your negative self-image.

Personalizing ● "Everybody at the meeting kept looking at me because I'm gaining weight." You tend to think everything revolves around you—a major distortion of the facts.

Either/Or Thinking ● "Either I get elected head of this committee or I'm a complete failure."

Overgeneralizing ● *"Nobody* likes me . . . I'm losing *all* my friends . . . *Nothing* ever turns out right . . . "

As you can see, depressed thoughts begin to sound monotonously alike after a while. That's because they *are* very much alike. For one thing, says Dr. Emery, "the chief characteristic of negative thoughts is that they're generally wrong." They're a distortion or an exaggeration of the truth. That's at least partly because they tend to be *automatic.* That is, they simply leap into your mind unbidden; they're not conclusions you've reached through reason and logic. In fact, in a sense they're not "thinking" at all.

How do "thought therapists" go about reshaping these negative, self-defeating, soul-saddening thought patterns? Not just by serving up a reheated version of "the power of positive thinking," Dr. Emery says. "In positive thinking you're replacing one global judgment (I'm no good) for another (I'm wonderful)," he says, and *neither* is realistic. As social philosopher Max Lerner has observed, "To believe either that everything is bound to work out or that nothing will ever work out is equally an exercise in mindlessness." The point is to put your life and your problems in a *realistic* perspective. Like a reporter, a scientist or a detective, you're looking to find the true facts of the case, to apply the principles of hard science to your own thought processes.

The plan of attack is in three phases, Dr. Emery says: awareness, answering and action.

Awareness: The First Phase

Vague, unfocused negative thoughts that lurk just below the surface of consciousness cause more harm than those that are dragged out into the open. So the first step out of the rut of depression is to become *aware* of what you're actually thinking and feeling.

Sometimes that's more difficult than it sounds, since these thoughts tend to be well disguised. Dr. Emery suggests using a sort of "instant replay" technique, thinking back to what crossed your mind just before a mood change or a physical sensation like fatigue, heaviness or butterflies in the stomach. Sometimes there *is* no preceding thought—you only later attribute a certain thought ("I'm worthless") to a certain feeling (sadness), says Arthur Freeman, Ed.D., a therapist at the Center for Cognitive Therapy at the University of Pennsylvania. "But whichever comes first, the thought or the feeling, we still find cognitive intervention effective," Dr. Freeman reports.

Another way to become more aware of your negative thoughts is simply to count them. You can use a plastic grocery-store price counter or a small stitch counter (sold in knitting shops), or just transfer coins (a penny is one thought, a dime ten thoughts) from one pocket to another. "These gimmicks remind you to become aware of your thinking," Dr. Emery says. "You discover that you have the same thoughts over and over again."

"It's important to 'concretize' vague, negative thoughts," agrees Dr. Freeman. "One of the simplest ways is to write them down. We try to help patients separate thoughts into three distinct aspects: what the situation is, what you're feeling about it, and what you're saying to yourself (your thoughts)."

Most of us don't consider situations objectively; instead we load them up with all kinds of projections and judgments, Dr. Freeman says. You may think, for instance, "I'm waiting for my girlfriend to call me but she probably won't because she knows I'm a loser." The first step is to strip away everything except the plain, simple facts: "I'm waiting for my girlfriend to call." Period. Next, you sift your experience in search of your true feelings. "The first thing you come up with may be, 'I feel like a loser,' but I submit that's not a feeling, that's a thought," Dr. Freeman says. "Then it's, 'I feel as if she'll never call' — again, not a feeling, a thought. Finally you get to, 'I feel sad.' Okay — *that's* the feeling."

Then you've got to tune in to your self-talk concerning the situation. Why have you concluded your girlfriend isn't going to call? If she's late, has it ever happened before? What other reasonable explanations are there to account for the fact that she's late calling? In short, Dr. Freeman says, you've got to *examine the evidence*. You've got to drag your negative thoughts into court, put them on the witness stand and confront them with the facts. Usually, they'll wilt under the pressure.

Dr. Emery, when counseling a woman who was depressed because she believed no man would ever want to marry a divorcee with two children, told her to go to the library and look up the statistics. She found that women with children were actually *more* likely to find new mates than childless single women of the same age.

Answering Negative Thoughts

Once you've identified and clarified the thought patterns that are making you feel bad, you've got to answer them back. One of the best ways to pry open the closed circle of negative thoughts is to learn to ask yourself good questions. Become a hard-nosed prosecutor and drill your negative thoughts but good. What's the evidence that I'm such a worthless person? Am I confusing a mere thought with a fact? Am I overlooking my strengths? Exactly what is the distortion in my thinking? Am I exaggerating or overgeneralizing? And so on.

A good way to clarify this process for yourself, Dr. Beck suggests, is to divide a piece of paper into two columns and write out a more balanced, fact-based, realistic answer beside each recurrent negative thought. A gloomy, lonesome housewife may think, "I'm neglected because nobody wants to be around me." But in the opposite column, if she gave it a little thought, she could answer, "Mary hasn't called because she's in the hospital, Judy is out of town, and Helen really *did* call, but I forgot about that."

Occasionally, Dr. Emery says, you may be so upset that no reasonable answer comes immediately to mind. So postpone answering—wait an hour or two, or set aside a certain time each day to write out your answers. One of his patients, expanding on this idea, created a "Wednesday Box" in which she deposited all the thoughts and ideas that bothered her during the week. On Wednesdays, she opened the box, tore up the thoughts that were no longer a problem, and tried to constructively answer those that still were.

Taking Action for a Better Life

It's not enough to simply answer your negative thoughts— you have to act on your new thoughts and beliefs. In a way, Dr. Emery points out, acting out your written answers to negative, self-defeating thoughts is a way of "reality testing" them to see if they're really true. How do you know for sure that you "can't" speak in public unless you try it? Or that you'll be rejected if you introduce yourself to someone you're attracted to? (It's possible you really can't speak in public, and you really will be rejected—but you'll never know until you try.)

For people mired in the deep mud of depression, Dr. Beck suggests working up an activity schedule, or weekly calendar with each day divided into hour-long boxes. The idea is to schedule something throughout the day, and keep a record of how well you did with each task—perhaps by rating the amount of pleasure or sense of accomplishment it gave you on a scale of one through five.

This simple little calendar can help in many ways. It gives you the true facts about what you actually do during the day—demonstrating to many depressed people that their lives aren't as bleak or empty as they had imagined. It helps you retake control of your life by breaking the rut of inactivity. And it helps you see clearly what gives you pleasure and satisfaction:

A Skill, Not a Cure

By becoming *aware* of your negative thoughts, *answering* them with a more realistic, constructive and adaptive view, and taking *action* to break out of your self-imposed trap, you can get control of depression and anxiety. But can you ever be cured? "Cognitive therapy is a skill-building process—we're not talking about cures," Dr. Freeman emphasizes. "Some patients call back in a year or so and ask to come in again for a kind of 'booster' session. But they've learned skills to help them cope, and their relapses tend to be fewer and shorter."

Do you need a therapist at all? "Thirty-five or 40 years ago, when the first psychological self-help books came out, there was a hysterical cry from the public and the profession alike that, 'You can't do it that way! You can't help yourself!' " says Dr. Reitman, a therapist who doubles as president of PSYCOMP, a California computer software company that's producing cognitive therapy computer programs to treat problems ranging from stress to sexual dysfunction. "But now we know that people have a great capacity to help themselves with psychological problems. And cognitive therapy, because it deals with thoughts, is especially suited to books, articles, tapes and computer programs. This is not *therapy,* mind you, but these things can really help, if people choose to help themselves."

If Your Child Won't Go to Sleep

If you have never been hassled by bedtime battles, wails from the nursery when you're in REM sleep, midnight nudges to "move over, Mommy, I'm coming in," bed-wetting, sleep terrors or nightmares, then you're probably not a parent.

Sleep problems in children, it seems, come with the territory. Frequently they cause tremendous worry, anger, fatigue and frazzled nerves. Your enjoyment of their childhood is diminished by your longing for the day they will grow out of it.

It doesn't have to be that way. Most sleep disorders can be corrected, usually in less than two weeks and without trauma to parent or child, maintains Richard Ferber, M.D., director of the Center for Pediatric Sleep Disorders at Children's Hospital, Boston.

"What is best for almost all children, after the first few months of life, is to learn to fall asleep in a crib or bed alone in a room that is fairly dark and quiet," Dr. Ferber suggests. "They usually will be better off if they are not held, rocked or nursed and if they are not soothed with a bottle or pacifier, radio or TV."

Sounds like seventh heaven, but how do you do it?

"Put him down while he is still awake," advises Dr. Ferber.

It's perfectly fine to rock your baby, sing him lullabies, read him stories. In fact, babies thrive on this kind of bedtime ritual, says Dr. Ferber, but put him in his crib *before* he falls asleep. That way he learns how to fall asleep under conditions he can reestablish for himself after waking at night.

What if your child already has a sleep problem that is turning night into day, waking his siblings and making a zombie out of you?

If you consult your pediatrician, chances are you will get

reassurance but not much help. "He'll grow out of it," "She's probably teething," "Let him cry," are the usual platitudes.

Dr. Ferber, a pediatrician who endured some sleepless nights with his own children, saw the need for more concrete help and made a study of the causes and cures of sleep problems in children.

In almost all cases he found that with a loving touch and a sensible strategy, most problems could be corrected in less than two weeks and frequently in less than one week.

Sound unbelievable? That's what Donna MacDonald thought. Her son Jeffrey would awaken and cry several times every night. Donna would pick him up, rock him or take him into her bed until he fell asleep, then put him back in his crib. When he was 16 months old, an utterly exhausted Donna sought help from Dr. Ferber. In ten days, Jeffrey was going to sleep without a whimper and hardly waking at all during the night.

"Dr. Ferber changed my behavior and gave me a strategy that worked," Donna told us. "I still enjoyed rocking him—but not to sleep. A little rocking, a bedtime story and a few hugs were part of the bedtime ritual. When I put him in his crib, I said 'Night-night, see you later,' and left the room.

"I let him cry for five minutes. Then I went into his room but did not pick him up. I talked to him lovingly, gave him a hug, then said 'Night-night, see you later.'

"This time I let him cry for ten minutes, then I repeated the scenario. If he was standing, I did not force him down. You do nothing that smacks of rejection. You are helping him learn a new technique. He needs love and support.

"Next time, the strategy calls for 15 minutes, then repeat."

Donna didn't have to repeat. Jeffrey was asleep before the 15-minute period was up. The whole scene took only 35 minutes. But sometimes, Dr. Ferber told us, the first session may take as long as two hours.

The second night, Jeffrey was asleep after five minutes of crying. The third night he went to sleep without a whimper.

There were several night wakenings over the ten-day period, which Donna handled the same way. Jeffrey is now sleeping through the night and Donna is enjoying her old vitality.

A slightly different strategy worked for Linda Logan,

whose baby was turning night into day. At 6:30 P.M., Matthew went to sleep without a whimper but with a bottle, and would wake at 2:00 A.M. ready to start the day.

To break him of the bedtime bottle, Dr. Ferber suggested offering one ounce less milk each night until there was only one ounce, and then no bottle.

To shift his sleep phase, Linda would put him to bed 15 minutes later each night. Bedtime crying was handled with the same 5-10-15 strategy used by Donna. In less than two weeks Matthew was sleeping from 8:00 P.M. to 8:00 A.M., and Linda no longer puts up with "jet lag."

Fear in the Night

Nightmares and sleep terrors—they both shatter the quiet of the night, but it is very important to note their differences.

When your child wakes from a nightmare, he is truly frightened and needs full reassurance and support. Stay with him. Hold him and let him know that you will keep him safe. This is more important than trying to convince him that there are no monsters in the closet. Even 13-year-olds appreciate this kind of reassurance when they wake from a scary nightmare.

After a nightmare, your child, if he is old enough, can describe a dream, but after a sleep terror there is no dream to report. A child having a sleep terror is not fully awake. He may cry out, scream, talk and moan all at the same time in a confused way. If you try to hold him, he will become more agitated and may push you away. When he wakes he will have no recollection of the episode, will actually relax and return to sleep rapidly. On the other hand, a child frightened by a nightmare will remain frightened and may be reluctant to go back to sleep alone.

At the time of a sleep terror, Dr. Ferber advises that you go into the child's room but avoid interacting with him unless he clearly recognizes you and asks for help. The child is unaware of your presence and may push you away and scream and thrash more if you try to hold him.

Sleep terrors usually occur one to four hours after falling asleep. Nightmares usually occur in the second half of the night when dreams are most intense.

After age six, sleep terrors tend to decrease. If they do

not, or if they increase again, emotional factors may be relevant and should be investigated. Should your child's nightmares or sleep terrors at any age occur frequently, work with him during the day. Try to determine what is worrying him and help relieve his anxiety. If you are unable to resolve the stress he is feeling, then you should seek professional help.

Help for Bed Wetters

Bed-wetting (enuresis) can be a child's most devastating problem. If, by age five, your child is still wetting the bed, it's not time to go after his training with more vigor, but to relax your efforts and try to remember—chances are you were once a bed wetter, too. The tendency is frequently inherited.

The majority of bed wetters are psychologically normal. It's the adults living with them who create problems by putting a burden of guilt, shame and anxiety on them.

Guidelines for parents of bed wetters include more don'ts than dos.

Don't assume that your child wets the bed because you have failed her as a parent. Don't think you could somehow have prevented it and don't use punishment, ridicule or shame in an attempt to stop it. These measures will not help, and they may prolong the bed-wetting and lead to worse emotional problems.

Make sure your child does not have a urinary tract defect or infection. Once you have ruled out these medical problems, consider that sometimes allergies are responsible.

In the treatment of more than 500 bed-wetting children, James C. Breneman, M.D., a board-certified allergist in Galesburg, Michigan, found that 8 out of 9 bed wetters were allergic to some food.

In these children, the bladder is the target organ, Dr. Breneman believes. The allergen causes the bladder walls to swell, thus decreasing elasticity and consequently its capacity. The subsequent irritation causes the bladder to contract, which causes voiding. The shutoff sphincter at the outlet of the bladder becomes swollen and won't tighten sufficiently.

Also, these children, because of their food allergy, are more likely to be fatigued and to sleep deeply, thus missing the get-up-and-go cue.

When offending foods are removed from the diet, Dr. Breneman has found the enuresis stops in a matter of days.

As the child matures, pelvic structures grow, enabling the bladder to hold a greater volume. Thus, at the time of puberty, even if you do not eliminate the offending allergens, the bed-wetting will stop in many instances.

The Right Attitude

No child, no matter how good his sleep habits, grows up without an occasional wet bed, a sleepless night, a frightening nightmare, a spate of crying in the middle of the night for no apparent reason. These are minor upsets that usually go away without treatment.

The most important advice sleep experts like Dr. Ferber have for parents, in order to keep minor problems from becoming major, is to help children develop a healthy attitude toward sleep.

The bedroom should be a pleasant haven, not an isolation chamber used as a form of punishment.

Don't expect your child to turn off his adrenaline like you turn off your car's ignition. Youngsters need a period of relaxation, a cool-down, before they can summon the sandman—a warm bath, a glass of milk, a story, a lullaby or just quiet talk about three good things that happened today and three good things you would like to happen tomorrow. This is a wonderful time for both parent and child.

Even with a bedtime ritual, every child has some nights when he will give you a hassle. Punishment, scolding and threats do not work. Positive reinforcement frequently does—a star for every night they go in without a problem; ten stars and they get a special treat, a coveted toy or a special privilege.

If your child stalls a great deal, you may be putting him in too early. Work out a schedule, then enforce it. Don't be wishy-washy. Consistency is the main thing, along with an appropriate bedtime ritual and supportive firmness. If you are lenient sometimes and firm at other times, your child will assume that this is one of the times when you are going to give in.

You have probably noticed that following Dr. Ferber's strategies means you will have to let your child do some crying.

Some parents who come to the clinic express the fear that letting their child cry in a room alone might cause permanent psychological harm.

"Not so," says Dr. Ferber. The crying is much harder on you than on your baby. Your child cannot understand what is best for him and cries when he fails to get what he wants. If what he wants is bad for him, you won't give it to him no matter how hard he cries, and you won't feel guilty or worried about psychological consequences. A poor sleep pattern is bad for your child and it is up to you to correct it. Expect him to cry during the retraining stages and don't be overly concerned, Dr. Ferber advises, unless he does not get his share of love and attention during the day.

Show your love and provide warmth and caring during the day and a little extra crying for a week or ten days will not hurt him in the least.

Environmental Health Updates

Beware of "Sick" Office Buildings

There's lots of glass, but the windows don't open. Interior space is "climate controlled," but it's often frigid in summer and balmy in winter. There are flower arrangements at many of the partitioned work sites, but a vague "new-house smell" permeates the air. The office is designed to promote efficiency, but workers complain of fatigue, burning eyes and sinus congestion. The imposing cage of steel and glass could win an architectural award but flunk a popularity poll.

If such features describe your own office, it may very well be that you are commuting every day to a "sick" building.

"Occupants of a building, usually large but sometimes modest in size, may complain of a set of symptoms which have collectively been named the sick-building syndrome," says Jan A. J. Stolwijk, Ph.D., of the department of epidemiology and public health at Yale University School of Medicine. "At other times it has been referred to as the tight- or stuffy-building syndrome." By whatever name, the problem is of growing concern.

The list of symptoms, which range from headache and sore throat to wheezing and shortness of breath, "is remarkably similar from building to building," according to Dr. Stolwijk. "Some people are severely affected by these symptoms, many more are annoyed. Unfortunately, our ability to treat and prevent the problem effectively is growing only very slowly."

High energy costs are a contributing factor. Newer buildings are tightly sealed and air is recirculated to keep down heating and cooling expenses. "Simultaneously, there has been a substantial increase in the number, variety and strength of sources of contaminants being introduced into larger buildings," Dr. Stolwijk says. "Chipboard is being used for sheathing and in furniture in large quantities. Carpets, curtains and upholstery consist increasingly of man-made materials, applied with adhesives—all of which release a variety of volatile organic compounds." In addition, increasing use of half-height flexible office partitions may interfere with original patterns of air distribution, lowering ventilation efficiency.

No wonder it's now estimated that up to 50 percent of the work force in North America and Europe is affected by sick-building syndrome.

Many experts are having second thoughts about the technological turn modern building design has taken. As one scholarly paper presented at the Third International Conference on Indoor Air Quality and Climate in Stockholm, Sweden, noted: "Contemporary energy-efficient sealed buildings serviced by mechanical HVAC [heating, ventilating and air conditioning] systems may be a failure . . . an anachronistic relic. In short, the time may have come to publicly question the reigning emperor's state of dress."

Yet something must be done for those structures already built. "Prevention is the best cure for buildings as well as for people," insists Professor Eystein Rümodahl of the Norwegian Institute of Technology. "But just as doctors must try to cure their patients when prevention hasn't worked, we must try to cure these buildings."

Let's take a look at some case histories of sick buildings to see just how successful the new breed of building doctor has been in diagnosis and treatment.

Diseases That "Drift"

"Critical parts of a modern building's air circulation system— such as filters, humidifiers and cooling towers—may spread airborne infections," says F. Marc LaForce, M.D., of the Veterans Administration Medical Center in Denver. "Cooling towers are used to cool water that recirculates in a ventilation system to cool air. Large fans pull air through the towers to be moistened. But fine droplets called drift enter the air supply. Such particles are so tiny they can penetrate deeply into the lungs. This drift can be highly infectious if contaminated with microorganisms." Legionnaire's disease, a serious and often fatal pneumonia, is just one of the diseases that can be spread by contaminated cooling towers.

Humidifiers, thanks to their ability to "amplify" contamination in the water supply and pass it along through the air, are also potential polluters. When investigators in England compared a 19-story air-conditioned building with a 6-story naturally ventilated office on the same site, they found a "highly significant excess" of humidifier fever in the tower block. Humidifier-fever symptoms include cough, fever and chest pain. To avoid such problems, Dr. LaForce stresses the importance of regular cleaning and disinfecting of key ventilation system components.

Infection was not the problem, however, when workers at a new, modern office building in the United States began complaining of upper respiratory ills and eye irritation. The building, which was designed for a high degree of energy conservation, had a sophisticated, zoned system for air recirculation. But what was being recirculated was formaldehyde.

Investigators discovered that the main source of the toxic chemical was particleboard-containing wood veneer on desks and partitions in the open-office arrangement. As the formaldehyde outgassed, it was not being adequately diluted and removed by the ventilation system. Increasing the amount of fresh, outdoor air mixing into the system helped solve the problem.

Sometimes a building may be only temporarily sick, but with devastating results. "One of the more serious problems involved a state office where shortly after the installation of carpeting, 20 of 35 employees were absent from work for a total of 521 hours," recalls Peter A. Breysse, Ph.D., of the University of Washington's department of environmental health. Complaints ranged from nausea, vomiting and burning eyes to chest tightness and diarrhea. When asked what made their symptoms better, 18 of the workers said "being away from the office."

"The ventilation system was turned off while the carpet was applied over the weekend," Dr. Breysse says. "So contamination from the carpet and glue was at its worst when workers returned on Monday morning." The carpeting was ultimately removed and complaints subsided.

Although air samples in this case did not indicate a level of contaminants high enough to qualify as a substantial health hazard, Dr. Breysse says, "There is no question that many workers have legitimate complaints that can be physically or psychologically damaging to health over a period of time." In fact, he adds, "during the past few years it has become apparent that office environment problems have reached epidemic proportions."

Trust Your Nose

The carpeting incident shows just how important a role our noses play in the sick-building syndrome. "Odors, especially unfamiliar odors, are a very significant factor in how comfortable you feel in any new surroundings," says Trygg Engen, Ph.D., of the department of psychology at Brown University. "The central nature of the olfactory system is that it's an arousal system. New and strange odors arouse and surprise, even if they're not unpleasant. They cause problems because they *keep* arousing us. They're there and they won't go away. For that reason, the best indoor air odor is no odor.

"Odors by themselves do not affect health. But our nose is the only indicator each of us has of the quality of the air we're breathing. It's not capable of chemical or medical analysis, but it stays activated until we know what the odor source is, or the odor is removed."

Documented cases of mass hysteria, Dr. Engen contends, almost always involve an odor that people were concerned about and couldn't do anything about.

Such lack of control is a recurring theme in sick-building discussions. "There is often a feeling among occupiers of such a building that they have lost control over their immediate environment," says Dr. Stolwijk. "They have lost control to the architects, the owners and the operators of the building. All the involved parties, of course, blame each other, which leads to general inaction. Occupants can sense this and they feel the situation is out of control. This psychological trauma may actually be more damaging to their health than the actual irritants in the building.

"Women will report discomfort much more freely than men will," Dr. Stolwijk points out. "So if you have a work situation where there's mostly men and just a few women, management may tend to ignore the women's complaints because they are the only ones complaining. This in turn will make them feel even more powerless."

The issue of personal control is underscored by the case of a large insurance company headquarters. The largest floor accommodates 400 workers in an open-plan design. The building is fully air conditioned, but only 10 percent of the circulating air at any given time is fresh from outdoors. Employees complained of headaches, lack of energy and other symptoms. Many said the air felt stuffy.

However, according to a consultant's report, "It was found that pollutants, bacteria, a lack of fresh air or anything fundamentally wrong with the heating, ventilating and air-conditioning systems were unlikely to be a cause of complaints." Some reasons for staff dissatisfaction that were pinpointed, though, included:

● frustration at an inability to control the environment

● a feeling that the environment was unpredictable

● a poor response to complaints

● a dislike of working in large, open-plan offices.

As an experiment, 12 workers who had complained of stuffiness were given their own small desk fans. Eleven of the 12 reported improvement in comfort.

While individual workers can't always regulate office temperature, humidity and ventilation rates, engineers and building experts have been working to set international standards for those vital factors. "In England in the 1960s, we started building glass-walled office blocks," says Donald A. McIntyre of the Electricity Council Research Centre in Great Britain. "As a result, we had severe overheating problems. There are lots of stories of prostrate employees being carried out to recover on the lawn.

"So we learned to set comfort standards, and to refine and maintain them. Then along came the energy crisis, and the whole emphasis changed to defining levels of *discomfort* that would still be acceptable to a group. What we found is that people start complaining about discomfort long before performance in an ordinary office is affected."

A Comfort Compromise

"The hard and brutal truth is we can't always afford to please everybody," admits Professor Povl Ole Fanger of the Laboratory of Heating and Air Conditioning, Technical University of Denmark. "People are not equal. Some like it a little warmer or cooler. They respond differently. Some people are very sensitive. They might, for example, require ten times as much ventilation as others to be comfortable, or they won't be satisfied. But that's too expensive, so we must say 'sorry.'"

Typical temperature standards, Professor Fanger says, aim at satisfying 80 percent of a building's occupants. The remaining 20 percent will be at least mildly dissatisfied.

"Institutional environments may have to be bland for the same reason institutional food has to be bland—for the widest possible acceptability," adds England's McIntyre. "After all, some people don't like garlic or chives on their hamburgers."

But dare we hope for more? "Someday I would like to see a 'gourmet' environment—a really pleasant indoor environment that makes your juices flow," he says.

Professor Fanger also has a vision. "Comfort standards are just minimums," he says. "What I would really like to see is more exploration of the positive. To draw an analogy with food, it's not enough to just avoid poisonous foods. We must follow the example of the great chefs who use their creativity to make some foods extraordinarily better than others. It is my dream that people will someday exclaim about the gorgeous climate they've just experienced inside a building the same way they now remark about the weather on a particularly lovely day."

SICK-BUILDING SYNDROME: THE WARNING SIGNALS

- Mucous-membrane irritation
- Eye irritation
- Headache
- Odor
- Skin irritation and rash
- Sinus congestion
- Cough
- Sore throat
- Shortness of breath
- Abnormal taste
- Dizziness
- Fatigue
- Nausea
- Wheezing and hypersensitivity

HOW TO SURVIVE IN A SICK OFFICE

What can you do if you know or suspect that you are working in a sick building? Here are some recommended steps you can take either as an individual or in concert with management:

1. Try to get people around you not to smoke. "This is often a very serious problem," says Yale's Dr. Jan Stolwijk. "Even if there's no one smoking in your vicinity, if the rest of the building smokes like a chimney, it's

(continued)

HOW TO SURVIVE IN A
SICK OFFICE — *Continued*

going to recirculate into your area. Campaign for a no-smoking policy."

"The most often mentioned complaints relate to smoking and stuffy air," adds Dr. Peter Breysse of the University of Washington. "Smoking either should not be allowed or allowed only in well-ventilated areas reserved for that purpose."

2. Check with management about the kinds of products that are being used for maintenance and cleaning. "Janitors tend to use the strongest stuff they can get because it makes their jobs easier," says Dr. Stolwijk. "You come into work and have no idea what's causing the irritation when, in fact, it's the cleaning that was done the night before." Usually those products can be exchanged for less aggressive materials.

3. Insist on reasonable comfort and ventilation standards. "Temperatures should not vary more than four to five degrees (70° to 75°F)," says Dr. Breysse, "and the relative humidity should be kept between 40 and 60 percent."

Better ventilation could reduce up to 75 percent of all office problems, he estimates. "Open-concept buildings need the greatest attention, since good air movement rarely extends below the partition tops." Raising partition bottoms approximately half a foot off the floor can greatly improve air circulation.

4. Materials and furnishings that outgas excessively should not be brought into the building. "Often this will mean getting assurances from suppliers," says Dr. Stolwijk.

Some carpets are shipped out by the manufacturer without being cured adequately, Dr. Breysse cautions. "We tell people, 'Before you buy a carpet, smell it. If it smells unduly strong, don't buy it.' You can't get much simpler than that."

5. If permitted, you might take a regular break outdoors. "Keep in mind, though, that this can actually backfire," says Dr. Stolwijk, "by making the problem seem worse when you return to your work area. The best break would have to be a long break, and that's not always practical."

6. Take some measure of control. "Generally, anything you can do that makes your environment feel better will help," says Dr. Stolwijk. "If you can get a window open, for example. Of course, that's often impossible. So I suggest that in situations where ventilation is inadequate, the person have a suspended ceiling fan installed. You can exercise control by turning it on and off as needed.

"One thing I don't recommend, though is a small, personal air cleaner. These devices are okay in a home where the air is relatively stable. But in a large office where air is constantly being recirculated, whatever little bit they clean up is immediately whisked away."

Donald McIntyre of England's Electricity Council Research Centre also mentions the interactive approach. "One school of thought in building design now feels that the more shutters, blinds, ducts, fans and other controls you can fiddle with, the better," he says.

7. Don't give in to despair. Dr. Stolwijk's own office is in a sealed building, but he reports relatively little dissatisfaction with his environment. What does he do? "I chase after the people who run these systems," he says. "That can really help if you keep after them."

How to Roll with the Seasons

Ever wonder why you can hardly stand the heat when those first 80° days hit in June, but when the thermostat climbs just as high on an Indian summer day in October you bask in the warmth?

Or why some people need an electric blanket on a cold winter night—and still wear socks to bed? And why they're always married to someone who likes the window open?

Or why colds and chills seem so abundant in the spring and fall, when the weather's changing?

We may not notice it until the fourth day of rain in a row

or a painful cold snap, but we're all affected by the weather and seasonal changes.

In some sensitive people, for instance, changes in atmospheric pressure or bright sunlight can trigger hormone and blood flow changes that start a migraine headache. Cold, damp weather can cause arthritis flare-ups, many sufferers claim, perhaps because it impairs blood flow to the limbs. And cold air can produce chest pains. It may constrict arteries and slightly thicken the blood, contributing to a seasonal increase in heart attacks and strokes.

"No one's going to say weather *causes* these illnesses. But for someone who's predisposed, it could be the straw that breaks the camel's back," says Simon Kevan, Ph.D., a professor at John Abbott College in Quebec, who has a special interest in weather.

It's true that you can't change the weather, but that doesn't mean you must be its victim. You could move to San Diego, where year-round 72° temperatures and low humidity create a near-perfect clime. "Every January we have a golf tournament that's broadcast nationwide," says San Diego forecaster Bob Dale of KCST-TV. "The next week you see pickup trucks with mattresses on top coming into town. It's people who are sick and tired of the snow back East."

That might seem like a drastic solution. In fact, you can stay right where you are and learn to live with the weather.

Heat- or Cold-Lover?

For instance, given your druthers, would you prefer hot or cold weather? And how can you make yourself more comfortable in both?

"People certainly don't hesitate to let you know their preferences for certain seasons," says Edgar Folk, Ph.D., a University of Iowa physiology professor who's studying the effects of cold on the human body.

The outstanding feature of cold-lovers is that they're carrying around their own thermal underwear. Their extra padding of fat is an excellent insulator, Dr. Folk says.

"At temperatures that make normal people miserable with shivering and cold, overweight people won't shiver at all, or even be uncomfortable," Dr. Folk says. But that doesn't mean you should stock up on fatback and cheesecake next winter. Weight-related circulation problems can make hands and feet vulnerable to frostbite, Dr. Folk says.

And fat can be a deadly addition in hot weather, because it can make body temperatures rise to the point of heatstroke.

Winter Appetites Crave Fat

What about the few pounds many of us seem to put on during the winter? Is that our body's way of weatherproofing itself?

Only if your exposure to the cold is very intense, says Dr. Folk. English Channel swimmers and Japanese pearl divers do develop an extra layer of fat, apparently in response to their regular exposure to extreme cold. And Canadian soldiers on bivouac in below-freezing temperatures chose a diet much higher in fat than normal. But most people's winter coats come from too much hot buttered rum in front of the fireplace, Dr. Folk says. We just don't need extra food unless we're so cold we shiver a lot or are outdoors all day long in heavy clothing, and then we need only about 100 calories' worth a day.

In contrast, summer appetites often wane. One possible reason: A study found that hot temperatures can moderately depress people's taste and smell sensors, which would tend to make food seem less tasty, so we'd eat less.

Exercise to Acclimatize

Exercisers can have it both ways. Fit bodies respond better to the stress of heat or cold.

People who exercise regularly develop a higher basal metabolic rate. They burn more energy all the time. This makes them more comfortable in the cold because their bodies generate more heat.

Does this mean they also suffer more in summer's heat? Not at all, Dr. Folk says.

"They apparently compensate with their sweat glands. Exercise improves and increases the ability to sweat and gives them a finely tuned apparatus to control their exposure to heat."

If your fitness activities take you outdoors, exercise some caution as well. In cold weather, warm up indoors first with at least five minutes of jogging or jumping jacks. Cold air causes the arteries around the heart to constrict, reducing blood flow to the heart. Warm-ups get the blood flowing to your muscles and dilate the arteries around your heart.

Unwind in Warm Weather

Use common sense in hot weather. Watch for faintness or rapid heartbeat, both signs of approaching heat exhaustion. Take the advice of weatherman Dave Barnes of WWL-TV in New Orleans, a city where 90° heat or 90 percent humidity are common summer nuisances. Save exercise and outdoor chores for the cool hours of morning or evening. Wear cotton, and wet your clothes down to stay even cooler. "My neighbor wears a wet towel around his head, turban style, while he mows the lawn," Barnes says. Know when to drop everything and go fishing. "Life in the South has a reputation for being just a little slow, and with good reason," Barnes says. "You just can't move quite as fast when the weather's like this."

Give Yourself Time to Adjust

As many runners know, given the opportunity, a healthy body can adjust nicely to either heat or cold.

People need to be outdoors at least an hour every day to become accustomed to hot summer weather, says Irina Cech, Ph.D., a University of Texas professor who's done research in heat acclimatization. This exposure stimulates the body's sweat glands to produce more, and at lower temperatures, so you stay cooler. Spending less than an hour a day outdoors will also help, but it will take you longer to adjust. And you have to continue your heat exposure, or you'll lose your acclimatizing response.

Regular exposure to cold makes the body respond better,

too, Dr. Folk says. Surface blood vessels constrict faster, conserving body heat. Less shivering occurs. The adrenal gland becomes more active, increasing heat production. Try to spend an hour or so outdoors each day in the cold, Dr. Folk suggests.

That's something Stephen Miller, a Presque Isle, Maine, meteorologist, tries to do. He cross-country skis just about every day of the winter, even when the temperature is a mere 10°F and the snow is piled up around his house. "It's not just recreation," he says. "It's absolutely essential to my physical and mental well-being. It means being able to get out, to not let winter get ahead of you, to not be intimidated by it." Miller also knows when to sit back and go along for the ride. "We work so hard here during the summer that I rather enjoy it when it gets so foul I can't go out. It gives me an excuse to sit in front of the stove and catch up on my reading."

Spring and fall are periods of unstable weather when the body has not yet adjusted to heat or cold and seems to be prone to illness. We miscalculate the weather and get stuck with improper clothing. We're in the midst of allergy season. All in all, it's a perfect setup for a case of the sniffles.

Sniffles, though, are the least of some people's concerns. Take spring fever, for instance. Some researchers believe that the lengthening days as winter turns into spring affect people's hormonal system, making them happier, more playful and more likely to fall in love. That's an interesting theory that has yet to be proved, Dr. Kevan says. He believes that at least part of spring fever's magic is that people simply enjoy being able to play and work outdoors again. "I'll tell you what makes me happy," he says. "It's being able to go out without having to put on my heavy boots."

But there's a dark side to this season. More suicides occur and some reports suggest there are more admissions to mental hospitals during spring and early summer than at any other time of the year. Why? One theory is that the same hormonal stimulation that makes most people happy may be excessive in some vulnerable people and cause emotional breakdown.

That's possible, Dr. Kevan says. But so is a sociological explanation.

"People who have been depressed all winter long become

even more so when warm weather comes and they see other people having fun. They feel alone, unloved and unsuccessful. In the winter, they can blame their troubles on the ice and cold. In spring, they have no one to blame but themselves. For some, the burden is more than they can bear."

December Depression

Late autumn and early winter also seem to be down times for some. "Not only are the days getting shorter, but up here in Maine that time of year is pretty cloudy, too," Miller says. "Everyone seems to get a little gloomy."

But those who get particularly irritable and anxious, and sleep more and more as winter deepens, may be suffering from what's known as seasonal affective disorder (SAD), a depression apparently caused by shortened days, which may affect the level of certain brain hormones. People with this disorder are sometimes helped by using bright lights in their homes.

Most people, though, are simply reacting to changes in lifestyle as winter closes in, Dr. Kevan believes. "Sure, I get depressed, but it's because I don't like driving home in the dark. I don't like having to put on three layers of clothes to go out, or being stuck in the house all night watching bad television."

Outthinking the Weather

The cure for December doldrums and other weather-related ailments, Dr. Kevan says, is to think positively and to change your behavior to foil the weather's attempts at control. Don't use the weather as an excuse. Get out anyway. Find good ways to interact with it—walk, skate or spend the day on the slopes instead of behind your desk.

"I believe that the psychological aspect of the human being is so powerful that it can often override any weather effect," Dr. Kevan says. "If you're happy, it doesn't matter if it's cloudy or if there's a warm or a cold front moving through. It's not going to change the way you feel."

And it might help you tune into the weather in a healthy way, not as an adversary but as part of nature's fascinating and endless cycle. Take a tip from the people of Seattle, who keep an eye out for that silver lining despite their city's heavy-duty cloud cover.

"We like the rain. It helps keep the air fresh and clean," says KOMO-TV weather specialist Ray Ramsey. "And when the sun shines, we all appreciate it a little more."

Surviving a Slippery Winter

The winter sun was barely above the horizon when Robert Sleight left his Washington, D.C., home for an early-morning appointment. A light rain had fallen during the night, and temperatures had dipped to just below freezing. Sleight hurried across the parking lot toward his car, eager to be on his way. But the next thing he knew, he was flat on his back, seeing stars, wondering what had toppled him. A moment later he realized—he'd been waylaid by a nearly invisible sheet of ice.

"The trick is to be alert, and I obviously wasn't," says Sleight, director of the Walking Association and chairman of the National Safety Council's committee on fall prevention. "I was preoccupied, walking too fast for conditions and not paying attention to the ground.

"The thing I remember most vividly is that I had absolutely no warning I was going to slip. It happened very fast, and because I was going backward, I couldn't really use my hands to break my fall. I was very fortunate most of the impact was on the big muscles of my shoulders. I was very lucky I wasn't hurt seriously."

Marvin Berman, of Exeter, Pennsylvania, wasn't as lucky. The 55-year-old truck driver was walking down a freshly snow-covered ramp at a delivery spot when he hit a hidden patch of ice. "I went up, and I went down, hard," he says. The arm he extended to break the fall took most of the impact. His shoulder joint was jammed so badly it's kept him from working for two years.

As their victims will tell you, winter slips and spills take their toll, and not merely in bruised buns and damaged egos. Each year almost 20,000 people die of injuries from falls. Many of these occur from November through March in the Northeast and mid-Atlantic states, and many victims are elderly.

And the doctor and hospital bills, days lost from work and lawsuits filed as a result of injury add up to big bucks. A simple broken arm can cost $1,000 or more in medical care. Using National Safety Council figures, Sleight has estimated that falls cost about $1 million *an hour* in the United States. With that amount of cash, you could encase every man, woman and child in America in a foot-thick layer of bubble wrap, and throw in a few skating lessons as well.

Even unconventional tactics can't prevent every spill. But Sleight believes many can be avoided if more people take a few simple precautions.

The Short-Step Shuffle

The same techniques beginning skaters use to stay upright will work for people who unexpectedly find themselves in a slippery spot, says Justine Townsend Smith, executive director of the Ice Skating Institute of America.

"Take short steps, always keeping your knees bent slightly, and hold your arms in front of you at waist level," she says. Your body weight should be over the balls of your feet and your arms should be providing balance.

Aim for the Buns

And if you feel gravity pulling, go with the fall. Bend your knees, tuck your arms into your sides and kind of collapse to one side, landing on the softest part of your seat, Ms. Smith says. As instinctive as it may be, try *not* to put out your arms. A stiff arm used to break a fall is often a fractured one afterward. If you must use an arm—if you'd otherwise fall flat on your face, for instance—bend it slightly to use as a shock absorber, Sleight says.

Bite the Ice

Eskimos wear mukluks, sealskin bootees worn over several pairs of socks. Oil rig workmen wear thick-treaded rubber boots. Penguins sport rough-textured orange flippers (or whatever matches their tuxedos). Practicality is the key to good winter footwear. Smooth-soled shoes can be as slick as ice skates, and high heels have the additional disadvantage of throwing you off balance.

"We recommend a substantial overshoe with tread," says Hans Grigo, the National Safety Council's home safety manager. The composition of the sole isn't as important as its surface texture. "For maximum traction, you want a thick tread that looks like a snow tire," Grigo says.

Such shoes work well on packed snow and help on rough ice, but on smooth ice no tread is going to work well. For that, you need metal cleats you can clamp or strap onto the bottoms of your shoes that can bite into the ice. Mountaineers use an elaborate version of these to climb glaciers.

Ice Breakers

It was still sleeting when Carolyn Kyra of Catasauqua, Pennsylvania, stopped for groceries on her way home from shopping. "I crossed the street with no problems, but as soon as I stepped on the curb, I fell," she says. Both bones in her lower leg were badly broken. "I have five kids at home and was laid up for three months, so this was a real crisis for us," she says. She lost her suit against the store because the law in her town requires only that people clear their walks within three days after a storm. "I think that's ridiculous," she says. "I think any time a store is open, the owners should be liable for a having safe passageway in front."

Most towns and municipalities have laws requiring that walkways be cleared within a certain amount of time after snow has fallen, so it's the responsibility of you, your neighbors and local business people to keep sidewalks clean.

Complain if you have to, Sleight says. "I'm amazed at how quickly they get out and clear the streets and at how long it takes for walkways to be cleaned," he says. "And sometimes the snow from the streets gets piled *onto* the walks!"

When you do shovel, don't forget steps and driveways, Grigo says. Many falls occur in these areas.

Shoveling won't remove ice, of course, so you'll need to

chop it up, cover it with cinders or sand, or use a de-icer. One study done by a chemical company found that the same de-icer many road crews use, calcium chloride pellets, melted ice twice as fast as rock salt and was even more effective at temperatures below 20°F.

Expect the Unexpected

The most likely scenario for a fall might seem like it should be a heavy freezing rain, where the entire landscape turns into a beautifully jeweled booby trap. But people expect it to be slippery, so they're very careful and avoid going outside if possible, says Walter Zeltmann of the International Weather Corporation in Brooklyn, New York. A forensic weather specialist, Zeltmann will reconstruct for court proceedings the conditions during a car, plane or body crash.

A more likely slip-and-fall setup is freeze-and-thaw weather, when snow on the ground melts during the day and freezes at night, leaving thin, clear sheets of ice on pavements. People hurrying to work in the morning, before the sun has had a chance to warm things up, hit these patches with all the panache of a tipsy giraffe. Add a light powder of snow to hide the ice and you've got the ultimate hazard.

Well, almost. Metal surfaces can surprise you because they freeze faster than concrete or bare ground. "Sometimes you see steel plates laid over holes at construction sites," Zeltmann says. "They usually have a little tilt to them. You hit one and it's like an unexpected ride on a sliding board. Down you go."

No one *plans* to fall, least of all on their own front porch, but it's best to be prepared for the possibility, Sleight says. At least exchange your slippers for a decent pair of shoes and put a winter coat on over your bathrobe. "Don't be casual about going outside, even for just a few seconds," he says. And use the handrail you should have on your porch and steps.

While you're walking, scan the surface ahead for glare, white frosted areas and "anything that doesn't look quite right," Zeltmann says. If you know where water normally puddles up around your home and in your neighborhood, expect to find ice there in the wintertime.

Keep your hands out of your pockets! "That's a very important thing," Sleight says. "Some people are seriously hurt because they can't get their hands out fast enough to break a fall. They fall flat on their face or head."

And try to keep your hands free to help maintain your balance. Use a backpack to carry items.

Winter falls can follow you indoors, too. Snow that drops off people's shoes in busy entranceways can create superslippery floors. Take your time negotiating these areas.

Keep these safety tips in mind when the north wind blows, and you won't have to be Mother Nature's "fall guy."

... And a Long Life!

A Medical View of Nutrition and Longevity

If you've read much about vitamins and minerals, you're sure to have come across books or articles about nutrients and drugs that are supposed to slow the aging process. It's a topic of intense interest—none of us is immune to the effects of time and we'd all love to learn a trick or two to stay younger longer.

Unfortunately, it's a subject that has produced a great deal of controversy. There are "true believers"—those who embrace without question every new recommendation that comes along. And there are old-line conservatives—those who insist no vitamin or mineral could possibly help slow the aging process or prevent its accompanying chronic disease. The subject has been muddled with irresponsible statements and exaggerated truths. Separating fact from fiction hasn't been easy, nor has finding a middle road.

But that's what Sheldon Hendler, M.D., Ph.D., has tried to do in his new book, *The Complete Guide to Anti-Aging Nutrients* (Simon and Schuster, 1985). The book discusses the latest scientific findings on just about every nutrient for which there's been a longevity or disease prevention claim. It evaluates each claim, pro and con. It points out promising areas that require further research. And it suggests how, and in what amounts, supplements should be taken, both by healthy people who want to live longer and by those with special needs.

254

We interviewed Dr. Hendler at his office in downtown San Diego.

"I wanted to systematically and objectively analyze the scientific data available for each of the micronutrients and other substances for which anti-aging claims have been made," he told us. "I wanted to be optimistic but critical at the same time—to present the good news, but only the news that can be supported by reliable scientific findings. And I wanted to call attention to things that don't work or are unsafe."

Dr. Hendler seems well qualified for the task. He has a Ph.D. in biochemistry from Columbia University, 15 years of experience as a researcher, a medical degree from the University of California at San Diego, and he is widely published in professional journals.

Currently, Dr. Hendler practices internal medicine and teaches at the University of California at San Diego. He also has a strong interest in the humanities. He played trumpet in New York City nightclubs to earn his way through college and graduate school, and wrote the original music for the BBC series "The Ascent of Man."

His move into preventive medicine wasn't just personal. It was professional and philosophical as well. "It was something I had been incubating for years," he says. "I realized that, in a very deep way, biochemistry really is the study of nutrition. Knowing how it works at the cellular level gives me a strong base of knowledge for using nutritional therapy in my medical practice."

The deaths of both his father and mother also made him painfully aware that traditional medicine seldom addressed the causes of diseases.

His father died suddenly at age 54 of a heart attack. "I thought it was a great waste," Dr. Hendler says. "At that time doctors were not thinking about how to prevent heart attacks." His mother died in 1975 of cancer.

"I had been doing cancer research for many years, but when my mother got sick, I suddenly realized how theoretical my work was. Here I was in a situation where my mother was dying of cancer, I was supposed to be an expert on cancer, and

I didn't know anything that could help her. I felt quite impotent about the situation, and I was determined to change that."

He found that the more he studied, the more convinced he became that medicine's real power lay in preventing disease.

"Becoming a doctor made me realize that many so-called degenerative diseases—cancer, heart disease, probably many dementias, certainly osteoporosis, emphysema, cirrhosis and degenerative joint disease—are all, to a very large degree, preventable. It also made me recognize that the therapies for many of these diseases caused more problems than the initial symptoms."

His education and beliefs eventually developed into the conviction that his own practice would offer the best of both alternative and traditional medicine. "I believe this is how every doctor will practice medicine in the future," he says. "I am hoping that through this book doctors will find they finally have something they can read and say, 'Listen, maybe there is some validity in these things, maybe we should start thinking about using them,' " he says.

One theory of aging-related disease is that it's the result of accumulated damage from destructive particles called free radicals, Dr. Hendler says. Some nutrients (called antioxidants) help protect the body from free-radical damage, giving them claim to anti-aging effects. Others act in a variety of ways. Here is Dr. Hendler's analysis of several nutrients with anti-aging potential.

Vitamin A

"There are literally hundreds of papers demonstrating that vitamin A can suppress the malignancy of cultured cells transformed by radiation, chemicals or viruses, delay the development of transplanted tumors and completely prevent malignancy in animals exposed to various potent carcinogens," Dr. Hendler says.

Supplementation with vitamin A has boosted immunity in some animals. And accelerated wound healing has been observed in animals given supplemental beta-carotene.

Some studies used large doses that would be too toxic for general use, Dr. Hendler says. "Vitamin A in excessive amounts can cause birth defects if taken during pregnancy and may cause bone disease in people with chronic kidney failure," he cautions. But beta-carotene has exhibited very low toxicity.

Niacin

"Niacin may be the best cholesterol-lowering agent available," Dr. Hendler says.

A recent study reported a niacin-induced cholesterol reduction of 22 percent and a reduction of triglycerides of 52 percent. "That's pretty impressive," Dr. Hendler says.

Taking 100 milligrams or more of niacin usually causes flushing and itching and can sometimes cause cardiac irritability and temporarily lower blood pressure, which may produce a feeling of weakness. "No one should take this much niacin without a doctor's supervision," he says.

Vitamin B₆

Of all the B-complex vitamins, B_6 seems to be the most important for normal functioning of the immune system. "It would be interesting to see if diseases with immune-function deficiencies, like AIDS, respond to supplemental B_6," Dr. Hendler says.

On the down side, there are probably quite a few people, especially women, taking more B_6 than they need. "B_6 is toxic in high doses and may cause serious nerve damage," Dr. Hendler says. "There is nothing in the data to even remotely justify dosages in excess of 50 milligrams daily for most healthy people."

Pantothenic Acid

This B-complex vitamin has a following among people with rheumatoid arthritis. "Evidence related to the claim that it prevents and alleviates arthritis is intriguing," Dr. Hendler says.

A double-blind study done in 1980 found "highly significant effects for oral calcium pantothenate in reducing the duration of morning stiffness, degree of disability and severity of pain" in patients with rheumatoid arthritis.

"Some of my own patients with rheumatoid arthritis say they get relief with pantothenic acid," Dr. Hendler says. "Clearly, more research is justified and needed."

Vitamin C

"Ascorbic acid is now being seriously investigated in leading research centers around the world with results, related in particular to immunity and prevention of cancer, that, though still far from conclusive, are very promising in several particulars," Dr. Hendler says.

For instance, a recent study suggests that vitamin C may provide potent protection against cervical dysplasia, a condition that predisposes women to cancer of the cervix, Dr. Hendler points out. There is impressive evidence that vitamin C blocks the cancer-promoting effects of nitrosamines. And there's some evidence that it can suppress the growth of human leukemia cells in culture.

Disease-fighting white blood cells have been shown to be partly dependent upon vitamin C for normal functioning, Dr. Hendler notes. And C may have at least mild antiviral effects. High doses boost the production and activity of interferon, a virus-fighting substance produced by the body.

Vitamin E

Claims that vitamin E protects against cardiovascular disease have been substantiated in the case of intermittent claudication, a painful narrowing of the leg arteries, Dr. Hendler says. People with this disorder who took 300 to 800 international units (I.U.) of vitamin E daily for at least three months required far fewer amputations than those treated with other substances or with placebos.

Vitamin E also appears to have anti-blood-clotting effects. "But until we have more and better information, no one can convincingly claim that supplemental vitamin E will protect normal individuals from cardiovascular disease," Dr. Hendler says.

Vitamin E is known to potentiate selenium's cancer-fighting antioxidant effects. And it may work alone in treating fibrocystic breast disease, a possible precursor to breast cancer.

"Claims that vitamin E extends life span have yet to be proved," Dr. Hendler says. One study found that although giving mice vitamin E lengthens their mean life span, it does not extend maximum life span. "The question of how much vitamin E is the correct amount for optimal human health and longevity is a very important one for which there is not yet an answer," he says.

Selenium

"There is no dispute over selenium's cancer-fighting, anti-oxidant effects," Dr. Hendler says. Population studies show that where this mineral's intake is lowest, cancer rates are highest. In animal experiments, selenium added to drinking water significantly reduced the incidence of liver, skin, breast and colon cancers. And selenium seems to be a potent immune system stimulator. Up to thirtyfold increases in antibody production have been found in animals given both selenium and vitamin E.

Cardiovascular disease increases as selenium intake decreases, Dr. Hendler points out. And there's been an interesting recent connection between a high-lead/low-selenium intake and the world's highest incidence of multiple sclerosis in an area in Saskatchewan. "It would be interesting to see if supplemental selenium affects this problem." (Since excessive amounts of selenium can be toxic, don't exceed a dosage of 150 micrograms daily without a doctor's supervision.)

Zinc

Zinc also appears to act as an antioxidant. And it's been found to be a potent immunity booster, Dr. Hendler says. "Research indicates that adequate zinc is essential to the development and maintenance of a healthy immune system and that aging is associated with immune impairment that can sometimes be partially repaired with zinc supplementation."

Other areas of study with zinc that deserve further research, Dr. Hendler believes, include its role in the maintenance of taste, smell and vision; in wound healing; in maintaining male sex drive and fertility; and as an anti-inflammatory agent.

Substances to Avoid

Not all the products associated with anti-aging claims work or are safe, says Dr. Hendler. Here are some he suggests you avoid:

Superoxide Dismutase (SOD) ● There is some evidence that, in injections, SOD can act as an antioxidant and anti-inflammatory. "But oral SOD is a big ripoff," Dr. Hendler says. "It is destroyed in the gut before it can reach the blood."

DMSO ● This industrial solvent may have antioxidant properties, but this has not been established, Dr. Hendler says. DMSO is being studied—but has not been proven effective—in a number of skin, nerve and autoimmune diseases. It does have FDA approval for treating fibrosis of the bladder wall. "No one should use DMSO without a doctor's prescription, and then only after checking that the substance is effective for your ailment," Dr. Hendler cautions. "The DMSO being sold in storefronts can contain contaminants and should be avoided."

Gerovital H3 (GH3) ● This is a 2 percent procaine solution similar to novocaine. "Claims that it can extend life span, reverse senility, increase sexual potency, overcome arthritis and protect against heart disease and nervous disorders have not been supported by scientific research," Dr. Hendler says. "Studies claiming these effects are mostly uncontrolled. Adequately controlled studies have failed to support these claims."

For those interested in a balanced program of anti-aging nutrients, Dr. Hendler suggests the dosages in the accompanying chart. The content and amounts are derived from his analysis of thousands of studies.

"The current Recommended Dietary Allowances simply do not deal with the maximization of life span," he says. "In no way are they concerned with the anti-aging or antioxidant properties of nutrients. People like us have to be the pioneers in this area. Within the next 20 years, authorities will recommend increased antioxidant supplementation."

Dr. Hendler also strongly recommends you see a doctor if you think you need any nutrients in larger amounts than those recommended.

ANTI-AGING NUTRIENT CHECKLIST

beta-caro-tene	20,000 I.U.	vitamin D	400 I.U.
		calcium	1,000 mg.
B₁	10 mg.	copper	2 mg.
B₂	10 mg.	chromium	100 mcg.
niacinamide	100 mg.	magnesium	400 mg.
pantothenic acid	50 mg.	manganese	5 mg.
		molybde-num	50 mcg.
B₆	10 mg.		
B₁₂	6 mcg.	selenium	150 mcg.
biotin	100 mcg.	zinc	15 mg.
folic acid	400 mcg.	iodine	150 mcg.
vitamin C	500 mg.	iron	18 mg.
vitamin E	200 I.U.		(women only)

Index

Rodale Press, Inc., publishes PREVENTION®, the better health magazine.
For information on how to order your subscription,
write to PREVENTION®, Emmaus, PA 18049.